a Rose from Two Gardens

Saint Thérèse of Lisieux and Images of the End of Life

Marcia Brennan, Ph.D.

Illustrations by Lyn Smallwood

Perspectives in Medical Humanities

The UC Medical Humanities Press publishes peer-reviewed scholarship produced or reviewed under the auspices of the University of California Medical Humanities Consortium, a multi-campus collaborative of faculty, students, and trainees in the humanities, medicine, and health sciences. Our series invites scholars from the humanities and health care professions to share narratives and analysis on health, healing, and the contexts of our beliefs and practices that impact biomedical inquiry.

General Editor

Brian Dolan, PhD, Professor, Department of Humanities and Social Sciences, University of California, San Francisco (UCSF)

Other Titles in this Series

Heart Murmurs: What Patients Teach Their Doctors
Edited by Sharon Dobie, MD (2014)

Humanitas: Readings in the Development of the Medical Humanities
Edited by Brian Dolan (2015)

Follow the Money: Funding Research in a Large Academic Health Center
Henry R. Bourne and Eric B. Vermillion (2016)

Soul Stories: Voices from the Margins
Josephine Ensign (2018)

Memory Lives On: Documenting the HIV/AIDS Epidemic
Edited by Polina Ilieva (2020)

www.UCMedicalHumanitiesPress.com

This series is made possible by the generous support of the Dean of the School of Medicine at UCSF, the UCSF Library, and a Multicampus Research Program Grant from the University of California Office of the President. Grants ID UCOP 141374 (2010-2015) and MR-15-328363 (2015-2019).

For my husband
Scott Brennan
and to the memories of my aunt
Theresa Glownia
and my parents
Joan and Alfred Gagliardi

With love to all

University of California
Medical Humanities Consortium
Department of Humanities and Social Sciences
UCSF - Box 0850
490 Illinois Street, Floor 7
San Francisco, CA 94143-0850

Cover Art
Designed by Virtuoso Press

Library of Congress Control Number: 2021948887

ISBN: 978-1-7355423-3-1

Printed in USA

Table of Contents

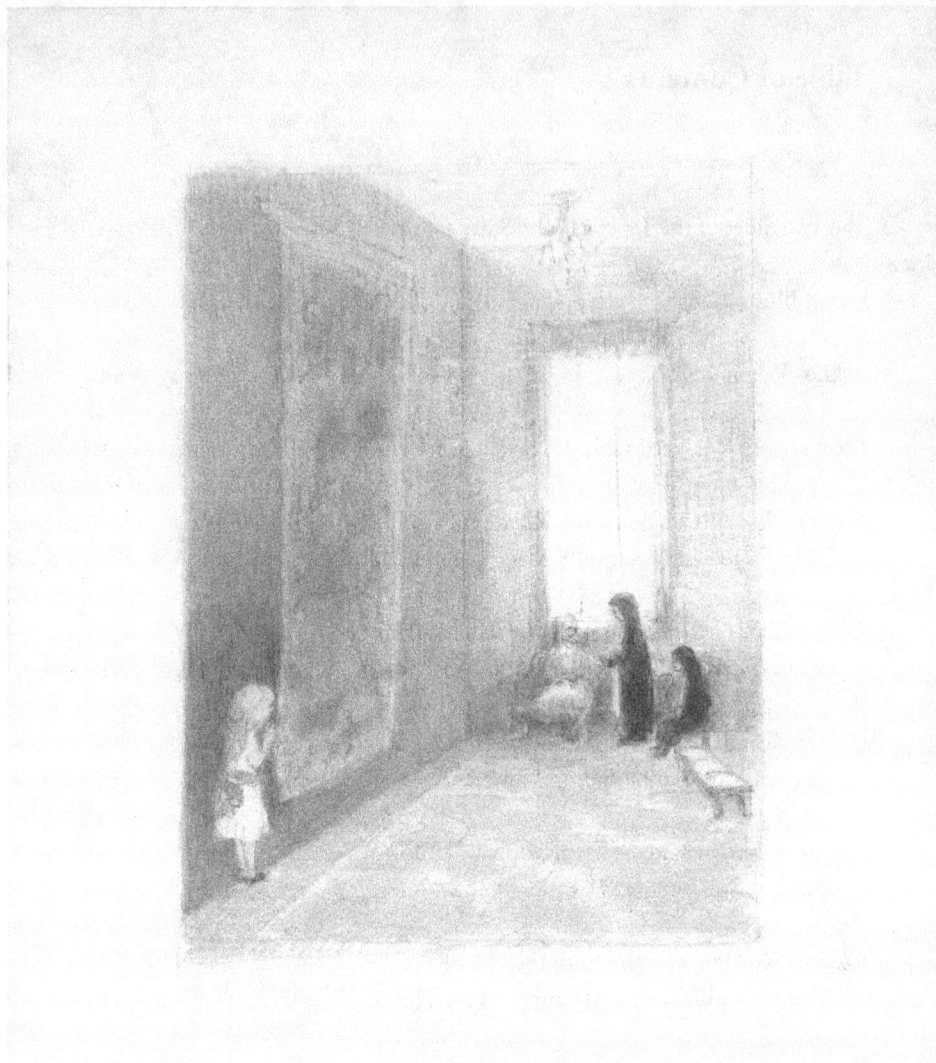

Frontispiece: Lyn Smallwood, *The Two Sides of the Tapestry*, 2016, graphite on white Arches paper

The Two Sides of the Tapestry: The Story Before the Stories

The middle-aged man lay in the hospital bed, rapidly becoming nonresponsive. He could no longer speak, yet he was still able to squeeze his wife's hand. The woman and I visited together for well over an hour to create a narrative honoring her husband. Later in the visit, she shared details of her own life, including a formative experience she had while growing up in West Texas. As a child, the woman and her mother regularly visited a cloistered Catholic Carmelite convent, and she became fascinated by an ornate tapestry that was displayed on a sitting room wall. This vivid childhood memory returned to her now, as she and her husband faced this crucial juncture in their lives together. During this transitional moment, the woman shared her image:

The Two Sides of the Tapestry

When I was a child, my mother would take me
To visit a cloistered Carmelite convent in West Texas.
The nuns did beautiful sewing,
And they made absolutely wonderful lace garments.

One time, I was in the sitting room.
The nuns were showing my mother their handwork.
There was a large tapestry on the wall.
On one side was a beautiful, bright scene
Of a man and a woman, and a castle, and animals.
But when I looked at the back side,
I wanted to throw up,
Because it was just a mass of tangled threads
In very bright, garish colors.
It didn't look like anything but confusion.

As a child, I would stand right at the edge of the thick tapestry.
I would look at the curtain flat,
And then I would look around the back
For as long as I could stand it,
Until it made me feel sick.
Then I would turn around to the front
And see the beautiful picture.

Our life here on earth may appear through a glass darkly,
Like the back side of the tapestry,
Where we don't see the patterns,
And we can't make sense of it.
This is like looking at my husband,
Lying there in his bed,
Dying of cancer.

But, God sees in the light,
And He can see the pattern.
Even as a child, I knew that the tapestry was speaking to me.
And, I knew it was God.

I later commissioned an illustration of this story (Frontispiece) from Lyn Smallwood, the West Coast visual artist with whom I had worked on two previous book projects. Lyn holds an MFA in Painting from the Claremont Graduate School, and she has served as an arts writer and critic for two Seattle newspapers, as well as for the renowned visual-arts magazine *Artnews*.

In this scene, a little girl in a party dress and patent leather shoes stands in the corner of a formal Victorian parlor. The child is dressed up for Sunday Mass, and she and her mother are visiting the convent following the church service. At the far end of the room, the mother sits on a sofa by a tall casement window, which allows her to admire the intricate details of the nuns' sewing. The translucent window opens up the scene while providing a luminous counterpoint to the nuns' dark habits and the surrounding enclosure of the convent walls. The delicate white lace of the nuns' handwork represents a point of contrast and complementarity to the bold, colorful patterns and the bewildering chaos of the tapestry that hangs at the opposite end of the parlor. Standing in the foreground, the little girl is nearly dwarfed by the massive tapestry. Gazing intently at the edge of the textile, the child alternates her stance slightly, so that she can shift her weight back and forth. Delicately lifting a corner of the fabric, she peers at the back side of the tapestry, while also trying to see the embroidered scene on the front.

As the woman later recalled, this experience enabled her to perceive a meaningful relationship between bewildering chaos and the larger patterns that formed the pictorial surface of the textile. This encounter allowed her to apprehend multiple possibilities as being simultaneously present and in dialogue with one another, a perspective that inspired the insight that familiar, lived reality is coextensive with an unseen spiritual domain. Now facing the end of her husband's life, the woman coupled these insights with an allusion to the biblical verse 1 Corinthians 13:12 ("For now we see through a glass, darkly; but then face to face: now I know in part; but then shall I know even as also I am known.") The woman carried this vivid memory with her throughout her life, even as the story became especially significant as she faced the end of her husband's life—and of their life together. Through this simultaneous engagement with the ordinary and the sacred, form and formlessness, vision and blindness, the woman received the strong impression that divinity was showing her the two sides of creation on a single veil.

Or, put another way, you might say that the woman was encountering a rose from two gardens.

List of Illustrations

Acknowledgments

Before all else, my thanks go to Dr. Jennifer Wheler, the founder of COLLAGE: The Art for Cancer Network, a nonprofit organization dedicated to providing innovative art programs for people living with cancer. It is under the auspices of COLLAGE that my work unfolds at both the M.D. Anderson Cancer Center and at the Hospital of the University of Pennsylvania. For the past several years I have been privileged to know Dr. Wheler as both a visionary leader and a wonderful friend.

It is an extraordinary privilege to work with distinguished medical teams. With profound gratitude, I would like to thank Dr. Eduardo Bruera, the F.T. McGraw Chair in the Treatment of Cancer and Chair of the Department of Palliative, Rehabilitation and Integrative Medicine at the University of Texas M.D. Anderson Cancer Center. My special thanks also go to Dr. Ahsan Azhar, Assistant Professor and Medical Director of the Acute Palliative and Supportive Care Unit of the Department of Palliative, Rehabilitation and Integrative Medicine. I am grateful to my colleagues on the Unit, including Martha Aschenbrenner, Chanelle Clerc, Stacy Hall, Thuc Nguyen, Ylaine Ong-Gabat, and Natalie Schuren. At the Hospital of the University of Pennsylvania, I would like to thank my colleagues Karen Anderson, Jenna Chrisanthon, David Cribb, Theresa Gorman, Michael Guzzardi, Krissy Hill, Mallory Jacoby, Joanne Klein, Dr. Hayley Knollman, Erin Lightheart, Jordan Mellinger, Jaclyn Rieco, Samantha Schad, Brianna Simons, and Jaelyn Walker.

My special gratitude goes to Sister Marie B. of the Archives of the Carmel of Lisieux, Lisieux, France. At Rice University, this project is sponsored in part by the Office of the Dean of the School of Humanities, and I am very grateful for the support of Deans Kathleen Canning and Nicolas Shumway. I would also like to thank Elias Bongmba, Chair of the Department of Religion at Rice. Just as this project spans the worlds of medicine, the arts, and the humanities, I am fortunate to have many gifted colleagues who have offered extremely helpful comments on the text. My thanks go to Travis Alexander, Melissa Bailar, Monica Bodd, Nate Carlin, Jose Chapa, Niki Kasumi Clements, David Cook, April DeConick, Jennifer Fisher, Dr. Deborah Franklin, Dr. Astrid Grouls, Julia Jung, Allan Kellehear, Anne Klein, Jeff Kripal, Lan Li, Dr. Kimberly Mendoza, Brian Ogren, Dr. Amberly Orr, Kirsten Ostherr, Bill Parsons, Gregory Perron, Paula Summerly, and Dr. Zoe Tau. I am especially grateful to Michael Olivas, the William B. Bates Distinguished Chair in Law at the

University of Houston Law Center, for providing collegial advice and counsel. At Rice, expert assistance has been provided by Amanda Focke, Diana Heard, Marcie Newton, Shelia Popillion, Jet Prendeville, Monica Rivero, and Andrew Stefl. As always, they have my thanks.

Lyn Smallwood has produced the illustrations for this and two other books I have written on the end of life. I could not be more grateful for her sensitive and skillful interpretations of these complex stories. It has also been an honor to partner with Brian Dolan of the University of California Medical Humanities Press. For several years, he has been a source of great patience and encouragement.

I have been graced with the friendship of Dr. Karen Cottingham, N.J. Pierce, and Dr. Julie Redmon. I am also grateful to have the support of my family, especially my sister Camille Gagliardi and her wife Dana Gillette, my nieces Kelsey and Devon Shay and Meg Elias-Gillette, my nephews Nicky Elias-Gillette and Aran Gillette, and my cousins Gene and Kay Bourquin, George and Clare Garner, Rick and Diana Glownia, Rob Glownia, Alison Healey, Virginia and Fred Larese, Nancy and Doug Tracy, and Elisabeth and Alec Zimmer. My husband, Scott Brennan, has been a source of love and inspiration throughout. I would also like to acknowledge those who are no longer here, including my parents, Joan and Alfred Gagliardi, my aunt Theresa Glownia, and my mentor, Pat McKenna.

Above all, I would like to thank the patients and families whose stories appear in these pages. This book would not be possible without the gift of their words.

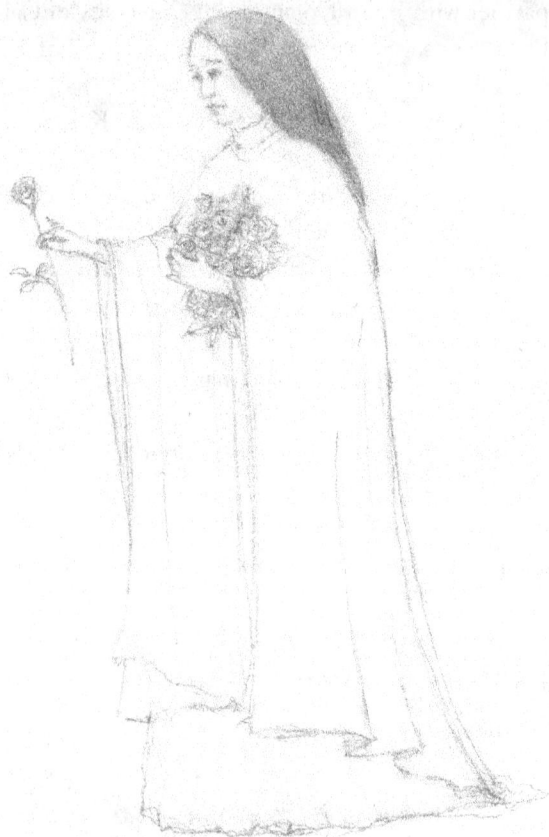

Figure 1: Lyn Smallwood, *That Rose Was Designated For Me: Saint Thérèse of Lisieux*, 2015, graphite on white Arches paper

Chapter One

We Need Lights to See Lights:
An Introduction

That Rose Was Designated For Me: The Story of This Book

On October 8, 2014 my aunt, Theresa Rose Glownia, called to tell me about a vivid dream she had in which she was visited by Saint Thérèse of Lisieux, the Catholic saint for whom both she and I are named.[1] Then in her mid-eighties, my aunt was experiencing various serious health conditions, all of which were very hard for her because she had always lived as an extremely independent person. At the time, she was grappling with the symptom burden associated with the treatment of multiple myeloma; ultimately, she would pass away three and a half years later. That afternoon, my aunt described how on some days she felt weak, with low energy levels and a spongy feeling in her legs. Yet the conviction in her voice was unmistakable as she related her dream:

That Rose Was Designated For Me

It was Saint Thérèse's day on October first,
And Saint Thérèse came to me in a dream.
It was some time between midnight and dawn.
She was carrying her cross with her, with the red roses,
And she handed me a rose.
It was a short-stemmed red rose, with a tight bud.
She didn't take it from her cross.
She already had it in her right hand.
All she did was look at me,
And hand it to me.
I think it was designated for me.
She just handed it to me, so gently.

And I mean—it was real.
She was there.
It wasn't really a dream.
That's the truth.
I could feel her.
She was so serene, so peaceful,
And I knew to have faith, that I was going to be okay.
I was just filled with serenity.
It was the most beautiful thing.

I've been seeing roses all over, even today.
Saint Thérèse was so peaceful,
She just handed the rose to me so gently.
It was the most beautiful thing.
I can still see her handing me that rose.

Shortly after our conversation, I asked Lyn Smallwood to illustrate my aunt's narrative. *That Rose Was Designated For Me: Saint Thérèse of Lisieux* (Figure 1) depicts Saint Thérèse carrying her familiar attribute of a cross surrounded by a cluster of roses. Thérèse's facial features display her characteristically tender gaze and gentle smile. The delicate lines of the fine pencil drawing form the sweeping folds of the traditional white cape and the dark veil that comprise the habit of the Carmelite nun. Much as in my aunt's dream, the saint appears to be standing in profile as she turns to offer the viewer a single, short-stemmed rose.[2]

As she spoke, my aunt's voice was filled with strength and joy as she emphasized how taken she was with Saint Thérèse's beautiful little smile, and with the tender gesture of being handed the rose. When my aunt heard her story read aloud, she almost couldn't believe the beauty of her own words. She then expressed her gratitude, and she gave me permission to share the story. Thus I begin this book with a dream that "wasn't really a dream," but a compelling vision of love that I have since come to call *A Rose From Two Gardens.*

While neither my aunt nor I knew it at the time, that conversation marked the beginning of this book. Hearing her narrative inspired me to reflect on the intriguing parallels that arise between contemporary end-of-life imagery and the themes expressed historically in the writings of Thérèse of Lisieux (1873 – 1897), the nineteenth-century Catholic saint who is popularly known as the Little Flower. Both Thérèse's writings and end-of-life narratives emphasize the transformational elements in life, just as they repeatedly engage the boundaries of knowing and not knowing, of representations and their constant overcoming. Some of the resonant themes include the paradoxical grandeur of small things, the spiritual significance of flowers, affirmations of courage in the wake of human suffering, the power of mystical dreams and prophetic visions, and vibrant conceptions of eternal life.

Yet at the outset, it should be noted that this book does not make a case for any particular faith tradition as the ultimate end of a "good death,"[3] nor does the text present a historical, biographical, or theological study of Thérèse of Lisieux. Rather than adhering to any particular interpretive tradition, I draw on the past for relevance and inspiration while offering new responses to the study of the spiritual. The clinical narratives are drawn primarily from my work as a literary artist at the M.D. Anderson Cancer Center. The hospital's diverse, multi-faith environment embraces pluralism while emphasizing an overall model of compassionate care. Because I live and work in Houston, Texas (and thus, in the Southwestern United States), many of the poetic narratives are voiced by people who identify as Christian. Yet whatever their point of origin, the stories shed important light on the ways in which people at the end of life envision a broad range of concrete and transcendent presences. Ultimately, Saint Thérèse's "little way" and contemporary end-of-life images emphasize the knowledge of the heart, which teaches how to see the hidden in everyday life, and how to recognize the dedication of love.

Inhabiting Multiple Worlds

In my "day job" I am a Professor of the Humanities at Rice University, where my teaching and research engage the fields of Modern and Contemporary Art History and Museum Studies, Religious Studies, and the Medical Humanities. Since early 2009, it has been my privilege to serve as a literary Artist In Residence in the Department of Palliative, Rehabilitation, and Integrative Medicine at the University of Texas M.D. Anderson Cancer Center. Since early 2021, I have expanded this practice to work as a literary artist with general oncology patients at the Hospital of the University of Pennsylvania. My clinical work is sponsored by COLLAGE: The Art for Cancer Network, a non-profit organization conceived and founded by Dr. Jennifer Wheler.[4]

As both a professor of the humanities and a practicing artist, my approach is informed by the insight that the words "cure" and "curate" share a common root, as both terms descend from the Latin *curatus*, which designates a person who has the cure or care of souls.[5] These terms apply to a curate, or "a clergyman in charge of a parish"; a curator, or someone invested with the responsibility of being a keeper of a museum, art gallery, or library; and individuals such as physicians who administer healing cures and medical curatives, including substances and treatments relating to "recovery or relief from a disease." Thus etymologically, a common bond unites those who cure and those who curate. In all instances, we have entered the domain of the caregivers.[6]

When I visit with people at the hospital, I record the narratives and images that are meaningful for them. Very often, I ask individuals to reflect on images that are close to their heart. Within this intimate practice, patients and caregivers provide the content of the stories, while I provide the practical means for the artworks' realization. There is no single protocol for our creative interactions. Because each person and each situation are unique, I allow the circumstances to guide the work. In this way, the encounters are characterized by a sense of openness, of not imposing a vision on others but of meeting people wherever they are. All of the work is done in a single sitting, and all of the words are the person's own. As I visit with people, I write down their words verbatim and then arrange the phrases in successive lines that resemble poetry. At the end of the visit I read the person's words back to them, and I invite them to make any additions or corrections that they wish. When I work at the bedside, I inscribe the narrative in a handmade paper journal, which the person is able to keep as a gift for themselves and their family. When I work remotely, I subsequently email people their story.

Throughout the narratives, poetry and prose appear as conjoined platforms, which creates a deeper and more cohesive sense of presence. I have often observed that, even after the poetic narrative is read aloud, it is still possible to feel the resonance of the words within the ensuing silence. Like the ringing of a gong, even after the actual sound ceases and recedes, it is still possible to feel the traces of a subtle presence as a reverberation in the air around us. How are the narratives able to function in this way? Notably, the word "narrative" descends from the Latin terms *narrāre*, *gnārus*, and *gnoscere*, all of which signify the sense of "knowing" that lies at the heart of knowledge and acknowledgment. These terms also relate etymologically to spiritual gnosis (*gnōsis*) and to diagnosis, which is literally a process of "knowing through."[7] While the end-of-life narratives present fragmentary and transient glimpses of a person's life, in these stories seemingly little things can convey important knowledge that might otherwise remain hidden. In so doing, the stories present a sense of the distinctive beauty that can emerge during this difficult time.[8]

It's Going To Be Beautiful: Encountering the Unknown

One day I met a lovely older woman whose room was filled with visitors. The woman was very weak and close to death; the medical team had described her as being "minimally responsive." Seeing so many people gathered in the room, I assumed that the woman would want to rest, and possibly, to visit with the friends and family who sat in a circle at her bedside. Yet as I was preparing to leave, the woman's husband became curious about my work and he inquired, "Did you say that you were an Artist In Residence here at the hospital? What exactly does that mean? Just what do you do?"

"Well, I ask people like your wife if there is an image in their mind of something that is special and meaningful for them, and as they speak, I write down their words and record them in a journal as a gift for the person and their families. It's always unique, and it's very tender." This brief description only further piqued everyone's curiosity. So, I turned to the woman in the bed and said to her, "Since they've asked, *is* there an image in your mind of something that is special for you?" The woman quietly smiled and nodded, so I took out my journal and started writing while everyone looked on in silence. Within a few minutes, I had recorded the woman's narrative. While she admitted that she did not fully know what lay ahead of her, she was certain that

It's Going To Be Beautiful

As difficult as this experience of cancer has been—
My image would be of the beauty of this experience.
It would be of a smooth transport
Out of this world,
And into the next one.

I'm not even sure what that looks like.
So, I'm just praying for a smooth transition.
I can't even imagine what that next world is.
But, I know,
It's going to be beautiful.

As the woman imagined the transition between worlds, her phrases evoked a paradoxical sense of knowing and not knowing, of saying and unsaying.

In such moments, seemingly simple statements can be extraordinarily powerful. The artworks can provide a practical medium for expressing this vision of something more, and a suggestive means for saying the unsayable.

I Wish We Had Lights: Recognizing the Extraordinary Within the Ordinary

Houston was at the very end of Tropical Storm Imelda, an extreme weather system that dumped heavy rain on the city and caused two days of cancelled classes at my university. By the end of the week, I was more than ready to return to work at M.D. Anderson. In the first room I entered that day, an elderly man lay in the hospital bed, actively dying. A person is described as "actively dying" when they reach the final stage of the dying process and they exhibit the symptoms associated with nearing death—such as changes in breathing, blood pressure, skin coloration, and orientation to the world around them. This man was surrounded by several adult children who were tearful yet filled with love and gratitude. Until recently, the man had been an active, outdoorsy person. His children described him as a rugged individual and a tender father who loved his family. As we visited together and discussed his life, one of the daughters described the special things that the man did around the house. Her words provide an apt metaphor for the themes that thread through this volume:

> *I Wish We Had Lights*
>
> *Dad would never just sit still.*
> *He lived with us.*
> *Just a few weeks ago, we were in the backyard together.*
> *I looked around and I said to him,*
> *"This is pretty, but I wish we had lights around the patio."*
> *And then, about a week later, I looked around.*
> *And all around the patio,*
> *We had lights.*

The woman's words contain a suggestive paradox, as fragments of everyday life become transfigured and they appear to be radiant. As the woman described the projects that her father completed around the house, she identified small things that are not small things—in this case, the decorative yet practical presence of the outdoor lights that would serve as both tangible and symbolic reminders of her father, even after he had passed away. Through these seemingly ordinary objects, the man would still be present, in another form, in the ongoing life of the family. His presence would continue as a subtle form of light.

While the imagery of *I Wish We Had Lights* is direct and concrete, my aunt's account of how *That Rose Was Designated For Me* conveys a sense of visionary consciousness. While the stories are distinctive, they represent two facets of a single subject. In *I Wish We Had Lights*, the ordinary and the immediate become illuminated and extraordinary, while in *That Rose Was Designated For Me*, the extraordinary is depicted in terms that are intimate and familiar. Yet whether the narratives overtly show or do not show numinous presences, they continually express the ways in which the subtle and the transformational become present within the parameters of everyday life.

Seeing Something More: Aesthetics, the End of Life, and Transformational Consciousness

When facing serious illness and the end of life, aesthetics can serve as a powerful means for expressing transformational states of consciousness. The narratives also provide a practical means to address larger ontological questions such as: How do we see, know, and find language for the part of humanity that encompasses *and* transcends the familiar forms of the physical body? These complex questions shed light on why I wrote this book and others like it,[9] why I do this clinical work, and why I teach related subjects at my university. As both an artist and a scholar, I am struck by the ways in which the interpretive tools of the humanities can be productively integrated into applied clinical and pedagogical settings to express a subtle language of presence.[10] Such themes are not only powerful on an individual level, but when approached collectively, they can shape larger cultural discourses on care, both in life and at the end of life.[11]

This is a fraught and timely subject, as death remains the capital fear of many—if not most—people, while the end of life often remains unseen and undiscussed. When people hear the words "terminal cancer" and "the end of life," they can become frightened and withdrawn, since beauty and hope are often the last things they expect to encounter at this time. Yet the artworks can be approached as gentle portals that invite people to enter, to be less afraid, and to help them remember what they see and how they feel. Whatever form the stories take, the narratives repeatedly demonstrate that it is possible to engage aesthetics to help dispel fear, ease suffering, and express insight. Again and again, the stories show that it is possible to go to the worst to find the best.

There Is Nothing That Cannot Be Seen: Maintaining Humanity at the End of Life

Like anyone who works in acute palliative care, I routinely witness extreme states of human physical, emotional, and spiritual suffering. The devastating effects of deadly disease take their toll in a variety of ways, from malignant tumors that protrude through open wounds that do not heal, to the often extensive array of invasive medical equipment that is inserted into, and extends outward from, fragile disintegrating flesh. Occasionally people cry out in pain or delirium, or they gasp for breath or hunger for air in the final stages of actively dying. Fortunately, the medical team can implement a variety of interventions that can help to mitigate these symptoms and provide comfort.

No matter how difficult or heartbreaking a situation may be, it is always possible to remain present and to see the person in the bed as a fellow human being. Again and again, I have seen that affirming a person's presence through narrative is a life-affirming activity that can shape not only how a person's life is viewed, but how we view life itself. *Thus I have learned that, even in the most extreme states of physical, emotional, and spiritual suffering—including those that arise at the end of life—it is possible to see the person in the fullness of their humanity. There is no one who cannot be seen, and nothing that cannot be witnessed, at this time. This insight is a gift for all of us.*

Throughout the visits, my attention is devoted to listening closely and being as fully present as possible. This allows me to take in everything and to acknowledge all that is there—including the suffering and the illness, the elements that are working well and those that are not working well—without allowing the pathological element to drive the conversation or the clinical gaze to determine the quality of the encounter. I also try to be particularly attentive to what the individual values, and the ways in which love, gratitude, gentleness, and a sense of spirituality can be as strong—if not stronger—than the experience of pain, grief, or fear. This humanistic approach not only allows me to be present to the person, but more importantly, this practice allows the person to be more fully present to themselves and to those around them.

In acute palliative care, I often find myself working with people at the very moment when the extremes of life appear at their most intense. As we navigate these deep waters together, we often discover bright lights shimmering up from the very depths of the stories. In the wake of great pain and suffering, grief and loss, we encounter scenes that are filled with love, joy, beauty, and gratitude. Again and again, while doing this work I have found that the lights are always there, but we need to know how to look for them, and we need to recognize what we are seeing. In short, we need lights to see lights. This book is filled with stories of how vision can inspire vision.

Legacy and Contingency, Doubt and Faith

These issues can be especially pressing when people feel a sense of doubt. One day I worked with a soft-spoken older woman whose narrative centered on her grandsons, whom she proudly characterized as "her legacy." While her love of the boys was clearly evident, the woman's narrative—and her overall vision of life—lay entirely in the domain of practical experience. When I asked the woman about her spirituality, she readily acknowledged that she did not know what to expect regarding the afterlife. As she said, "I wish I had a strong faith that could help me accept what comes next. I'm struggling to understand what comes after life." While the woman courageously acknowledged her own vulnerability and her sense of not knowing, her spiritual uncertainty was causing her a great deal of pain and fear. All I could do was to remind her of the sacredness of the love that she felt—and that she would always feel—for her grandsons.

In contrast, on another day I worked with a middle-aged woman who was very close to the end of her life. Communicating remotely through Zoom, the woman told me all about her children, and she shared many details of their lives. At the end of the visit, she linked her love of her children with her strong spiritual faith, both of which she saw as expressions of the continuity of life and love:

I feel my children are the best part of me.
I feel my kids are a reflection of who I am.
My faith is also very important.
I believe strongly in the power of prayer.
I truly believe that prayer changes things.
I want my kids to know that faith doesn't cost you anything to have.
When you have nothing,
You have your faith to confide in,
To cling to,
And to hold onto.

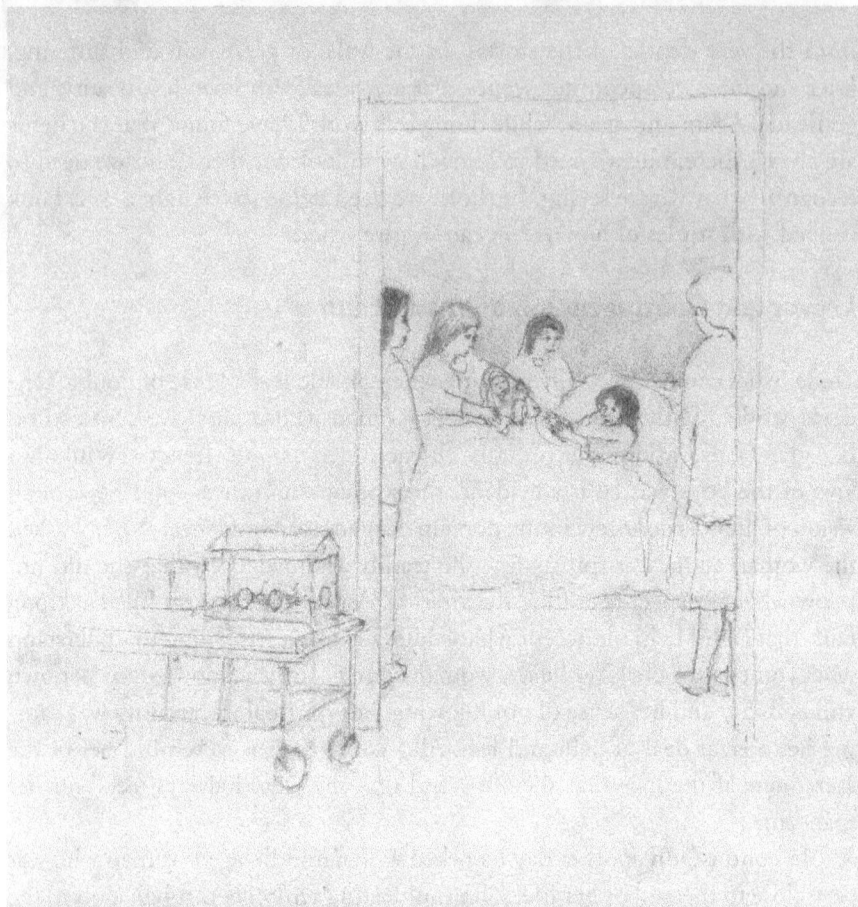

Figure 2: Lyn Smallwood, *He Might Have Been Looking at Me,* 2020, graphite on white Strathmore drawing paper

And, I feel like—
No matter who you are—
Love is the one thing that matters,
To us all.

Interweaving her love for her children with her strong spiritual faith, this woman consciously acknowledged how one presence connects with another. As she reflected on "the best part of me," she evoked the ways in which the bonds of love, faith, and presence would continue on with a life of their own, one that extended well beyond the finite boundaries of a human lifetime.

He Might Have Been Looking at Me: Endings and Beginnings

One day I saw something that, in all my years in palliative care, I had never seen before. In fact, *no one* had ever seen anything quite like this before. An incubator was wheeled over on a gurney from a neighboring children's hospital with a tiny, premature baby inside. The baby's mother was a patient on our Unit. While she was not yet actively dying, the woman was minimally oriented and she could no longer speak. Ultimately, she would pass away about two weeks later.

On the day of the visit, I was given some background information on the case. After the baby had been delivered several months early by C-section, the mother wasn't doing well and, due to her advanced cancer, she never left the hospital. Yet even as the woman faced the end of her life, that day was the first and only time she would ever see her son. During the visit, the sleeping baby opened his eyes just once, and she opened her eyes, as well. The experience was extremely touching, and both the family and the staff were moved to tears. I kept thinking to myself: How many times in a person's life would they ever get to witness such a remarkable sight?

Before the baby arrived, I visited with the family to create a tribute to the woman, then I stepped out of the crowded room. As I stood at the Nurse's Station writing up the narrative, the baby was wheeled over from the Neonatal Intensive Care Unit (NICU) of the neighboring hospital. The baby arrived in an incubator, which was placed on a gurney and accompanied by three NICU nurses. While working in palliative care, I have seen gurneys on our floor many times after someone has passed away and the attendants arrive to bring the body to the morgue. Yet I had never seen an incubator on a gurney. This sight filled my eyes with tears. Outside the woman's door, several of the nurses, physicians, and aides stood around the room, forming a ring. Many of us were crying because we knew that this would be the first and only time that the mother and son would ever see one another. The baby was very good throughout the visit, not even crying once. After everyone left, I asked the father what he thought of the experience. He said:

> *That was wonderful, wonderful, very wonderful.*
> *My wife got what she wanted.*
> *Thank God.*
> *It wouldn't have been possible without the social worker and the nurses.*
>
> *He's my one boy, and my last child.*
> *During the visit he opened his eyes.*
> *He might have been looking at me.*

Lyn Smallwood's pencil drawing (Figure 2) depicts the moment when, as the woman faced the end of her life, she got to see her son at the beginning of his. In this intimate scene, the family is framed in the hospital doorway, while the empty incubator sits on a gurney just outside the door. Within the room the dying woman is surrounded by her family, while a nurse holds the baby up for his mother to see, so that she can touch his little foot. Unfolding along the extreme edges of life itself, the structure of this story is chiasmatic, as openings and closings, births and deaths, beginnings and ends create a conjunction—and they meet in a place of oneness. That day I was able to witness the moment when this philosophical and spiritual pattern assumed living form, when their eyes briefly met and opposites folded back on one another in a state of mutual recognition. For all of us who were fortunate enough to be present at that moment, we witnessed a fragile yet powerful scene that will be with us for the rest of our lives.

Like many of the stories that fill this volume, the trajectory of *He Might Have Been Looking at Me* is circular rather than linear. Much like the wheels turning on the gurney that brought the infant to his mother, this story contains a sense of both turning and overturning familiar expectations. Multiple pathways come full circle as ends meet beginnings and people feel a sense of completion. If I were to phrase this in technical terms, I would say that such stories exemplify a striking coincidence of opposites (*coincidentia oppositorum*), a paradoxical sense of circularity that evokes opposites that are not opposites but two facets of a single state of being. When witnessing such scenes, we find ourselves encountering a rose from two gardens.

Conjoining Multiple Worlds: Audience and Readership

By engaging these subjects, *A Rose From Two Gardens* contributes to the literatures of medicine, the arts, and the humanities as it links the practical insights of the clinical domain with subtle themes of sacrality, grace, and nondual presence. This multilayered approach can help to integrate the tools and methods of literary aesthetics, Religious Studies, and the Medical Humanities into applied clinical domains. Throughout the text, the poetic narratives appear in italicized type. The book features over eighty original literary artworks and thirty accompanying illustrations. The artworks can provide a practical means to envision the conjunction of the ordinary and the extraordinary, the concrete and the subtle, the familiar and the transcendent. In so doing, the words and images can change not only how we view the end of life, but also how we view life itself—and thus, how we actively live our lives.

A Rose From Two Gardens will be of interest to medical, academic, and general audiences. Just as the book is a hybrid volume that is composed of both primary and secondary texts, the stories feature a strong emotional component. This is a teaching volume whose lessons are learned by opening the eyes, the mind, and the heart. Just as the book examines the various ways in which aesthetics can be integrated into the clinical setting, the text will appeal to healthcare professionals who seek to incorporate humanistic knowledge into the theory and practice of medicine. In a report on *The Fundamental Role of the Arts and Humanities in Medical Education*, the Association of American Medical Colleges has noted:

> Now more than ever, physicians must learn to interweave their developing scientific knowledge with emotional intelligence, critical thinking skills, and an understanding of social context. The integration of the arts and humanities into medicine and medical education may be essential to educating a physician workforce that can effectively contribute to optimal health care outcomes for patients and communities.[12]

In Chapter Three I discuss some of the specific responses that this work has generated from medical and pre-medical audiences. Here I will note that the clinical readership can include not only physicians and nurses—especially those working in the fields of palliative and geriatric care, public health, internal medicine, and chronic pain—but also hospital chaplains and other spiritual caregivers, psychologists, counselors, social workers, expressive arts therapists, and medical students. This book will also be of interest to practicing artists and to academic readers in the fields of Cultural Studies, the Medical Humanities, Narrative Medicine, literary creativity, Expressive Arts Therapies, and Religious Studies. Ultimately, this book is for everyone who is drawn to it, including people who just want to read the stories.

This work has repeatedly shown me the ways in which humanistic interpretative tools can be aptly suited for collaborations with nontraditional subjects, particularly those that expand the reach of the humanities into difficult areas of modern life. Yet some of the issues this work raises are methodologically complex. During the clinical visits, the subjects we discuss are often so intense and nuanced as to be "off the charts," and thus, they do not readily lend themselves to quantitative study or data-driven assessment metrics.[13] These methodological issues speak at once to the distinctive value, and to some of the complications, associated with integrating qualitative and humanistic approaches into a medical context. In such sensitive clinical settings—as in life itself—how do we begin to see what ordinarily cannot be seen, and hear what ordinarily cannot be heard? Again and again, the poetic narratives express the ineffable and hold the unholdable, while anchoring these delicate and powerful visions within the clarity of everyday life and language.

When commenting on related themes that arise at the end of life, Dr. David Casarett has observed that the issues that are greatly valued by patients—yet which are seldom captured in the data collected by healthcare institutions—include "emotional and spiritual support" and "respect for dignity." Attending to these concerns can allow patients and caregivers to feel a greater "sense of dignity and control."[14] While individuals facing the end of life tend to value personalized compassionate care, these themes are not necessarily reflected in the institutional metrics that assess quality of care. A *Lancet Oncology* Commission has similarly advocated adopting a multidisciplinary approach that integrates oncology and palliative care. The Commission enumerates the many benefits of combining paradigms for achieving the goals of patient-centered care, while noting that some of the barriers to this model concern "the common misconception that palliative care is end-of-life care only, stigmatization of death and dying, and insufficient infrastructure and funding."[15] My experiences have repeatedly shown me that, by prioritizing and enhancing the quality of life, palliative care represents an affirmation of life itself, one that simultaneously bears on how we care for the dying *and* for the living.

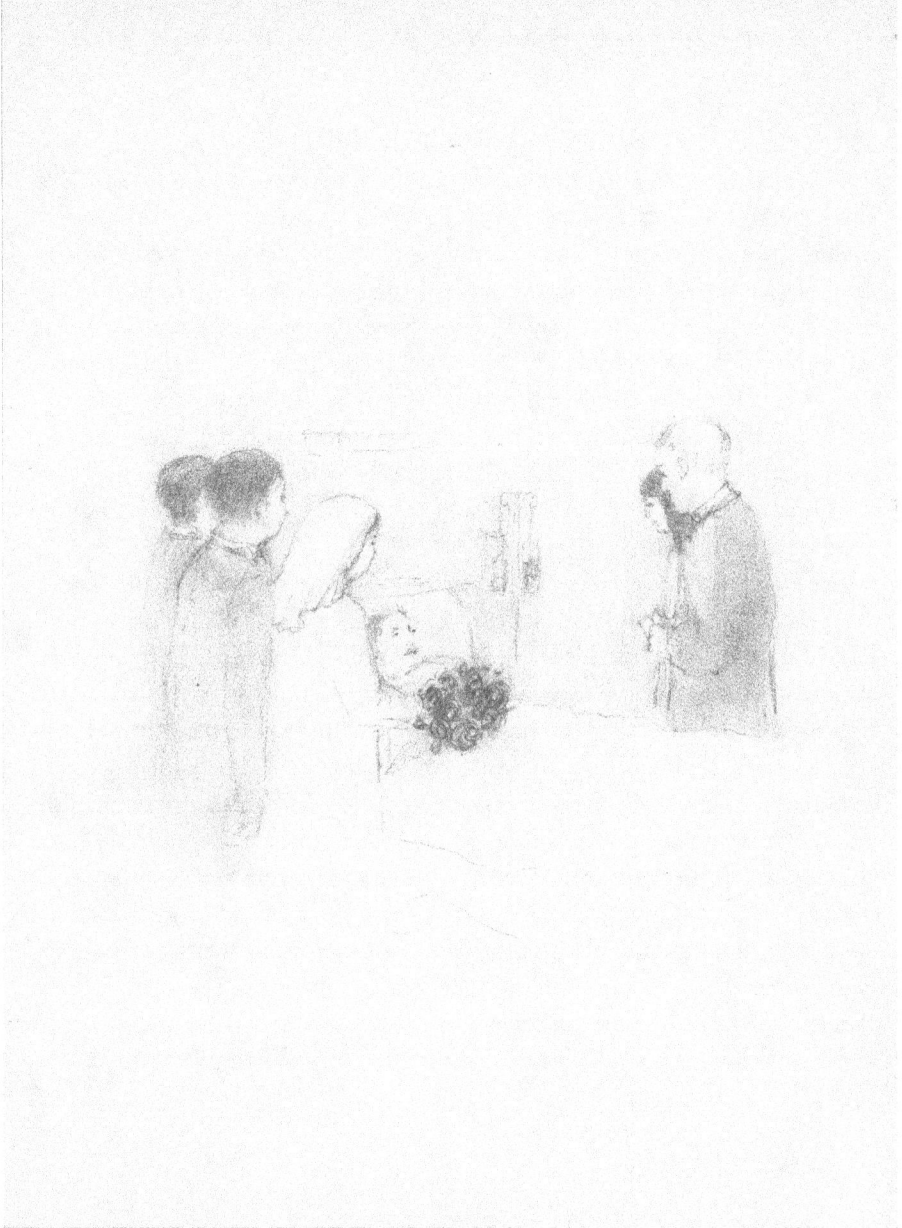

Figure 3: Lyn Smallwood, *In Peace with God*, 2020, graphite on white Strathmore drawing paper

We Can't Put This Into Words: Seeing the Otherwise Unseen

One afternoon I both witnessed and participated in a remarkable event—a wedding that was performed at the very end of life. In all my years working in palliative care, I have only observed such an event a handful of times. This ceremony involved a couple in which the groom was a middle-aged, Spanish-speaking man with advanced lung cancer. Due to his severe dyspnea, communication was very difficult, and the man was connected to a high-flow oxygen device as well as to several IV bags that dispensed both pain medication and antibiotics. When I initially arrived on the Palliative Care Unit that day, I asked the charge nurse when the wedding would take place. To my surprise, she responded, "Any minute now. As soon as the Catholic priest arrives." Knowing how important this event would be for the man and his family, I went into this room first, so that I could record the narrative as an end of life wedding gift for them.

The timing was perfect. While the man spoke softly about his family background, his two adult sons served as translators. During our brief visit, I learned that the man and his wife had been legally married for several decades but that they had never had a church wedding. Then the priest arrived. After brief introductions, the priest asked if, as a non-family member, I would consent to remain and serve as a witness to the marriage. I told him that I would be honored to do so. As the priest conducted the wedding service in Spanish, the woman stood at her husband's bedside with her head covered by a simple veil, and a bouquet of crimson roses in her hands. After the ceremony concluded, I asked the family about this experience, and the eldest son translated the poetic narrative for his parents. The man broke into tears as he spoke, as the subject was so close to all of their hearts. Much like the vows that the couple exchanged, the artwork conjoined the man's and the woman's voices together within a single narrative as they told a story of being:

In Peace with God

We're married for many years,
But getting married in the church
Is one of the things we've always dreamed of.
That has been important, whenever we talk about it.
But it never happened in the church.
Still, it has been one of our dreams.

This is important because—
It has always been a life dream to us—
Even at this time.
That way, we can both be
In peace with God.

We can't put this into words.

When I write about my hospital experiences, information such as patient names and dates are omitted or generalized in order to render the subjects anonymous. Yet because the specific date of the wedding was such an important feature of the narrative, the family kindly granted permission to share this aspect of the story. This wedding took place on January 2nd, which is Saint Thérèse's birthday. On that particular year, the date fell on a day that is not my typical day to be working at the hospital. Knowing that it can be exceptionally difficult for people to face the end of life during the holiday season, I decided to visit the Palliative Care Unit the day after New Year's, to see if anyone would like to work together. All of which is to say that this visit was not supposed to have happened at all, since it wasn't my day to be on the Unit, let alone to arrive just a few moments before a priest came in to perform a wedding ceremony that fulfilled a couple's life dream at the end of their life together. To this day, I remain extremely grateful for the coincidence of the timing, which allowed me to be present to serve as both a witness and an artist, to record an end-of-life wedding that took place on Saint Thérèse's birthday.

The couple's narrative vividly expresses the complex sense of love and spirituality that can arise when people confront a situation that exceeds the limits of language. Just as the details of the wedding scene are clearly recognizable, the narrative provides a vehicle for imagining the unimaginable. *In Peace with God* recounts a couple's realization of a dream that unfolded at the very edges of life and language. Just as they affirmed their bonds of commitment through the exchange of vows, when the couple tried to describe the significance that this event held for them, they concluded, "We can't put this into words." In so doing, their story provides insight into how people manage to say what cannot be said, and how we picture what cannot ever be fully pictured.

Resonating with these themes, Lyn Smallwood's illustration (Figure 3) presents an intimate view of this scene, as if the spectator stands poised in the doorway. A man lies in a hospital bed at the end of life, with several IV bags hanging at his side. His wife and two adult sons encircle him on one side, while the Catholic priest and I stand at the opposite side of the bed. The priest holds a prayer book, while the woman wears a simple white veil and she holds a lush bouquet of roses in her hands. The textured pencil lines of the drawing create a soft atmosphere, much like the ambience that filled the room. As I stood witnessing this dreamlike scene, I noticed that the red roses had tiny bits of gold at their centers. Expressing a delicate yet powerful sense of transformation, this narrative sheds light on the unseen depths that lay hidden within the familiar details of life itself—much like the gold that lay sheltered at the center of the crimson roses that the woman held so tenderly in her hands.

Notes

1. Regarding this story, see my book *Put It On the Windowsill: An Italian-American Family Memoir* (Staffordshire, UK: Dark River, 2019), 151–56.

2. This story represents a striking example of what the historian of religion Robert Orsi has characterized, in another context, as an intimate history in which "family dynamics are one spring of sacred presences." In such narratives, spirituality unfolds within "experience and practice, in relationships between heaven and earth, in the circumstances of people's lives and histories, and in the stories people tell about them." See Robert A. Orsi, *Between Heaven and Earth: The Religious Worlds People Make and the Scholars Who Study Them* (Princeton: Princeton University Press, 2005), 13, 18. In a subsequent volume, Orsi identifies what he calls an unfixed boundary between the realms of the living and the dead, and he notes that many Catholics believe that loved ones and supernatural figures accompany individuals at the end of life. See Robert A. Orsi, *History and Presence* (Cambridge: Harvard University Press, 2016).

3. For a different perspective on end of life imagery, see James W. Green, *Beyond the Good Death: The Anthropology of Modern Dying* (Philadelphia: University of Pennsylvania Press, 2008), 25–30. As an anthropologist, Green characterizes various end-of-life activities as forms of mythopraxis, in which people serve as agents of their own mythologies. In this volume Green writes extensively about our contemporary society and the many venues in which the sacred is made real through the connections between the everyday and the mysterious realms.

4. For information on the nonprofit organization COLLAGE: The Art for Cancer Network, see https://www.collageartforcancer.org/.

5. See the entries on "cure" and "curate" in the *Oxford English Dictionary*, 2nd ed. (Oxford: Clarendon Press, 1989), and in *Webster's Seventh New Collegiate Dictionary* (Springfield, MA: Merriam, 1969), 203.

6. As this suggests, the subject of care relates to the philosophical tradition of the *cura*, the ancient caregiving and caretaking practices of concern, solicitude, and responsibility that link the practical details of life experience to larger conceptions of the life of the soul. On these themes, see Jacques Derrida, *The Gift of Death*, 2nd ed., trans. David Wills (Chicago: University of Chicago Press, 2008), 14–15.

7. See the entry on "*gnō*" (or knowledge) that lies at the root of "narrative" in Calvert Watkins, ed., *The American Heritage Dictionary of Indo-European Roots*, 2nd ed. (Boston: Houghton Mifflin, 2000), 32–33. See also the entries on "gnosis" and "narrate" in *Webster's Seventh New Collegiate Dictionary*, 356, 562.

8. Regarding the ways in which this work differs from Rita Charon's practice of narrative medicine, see my book *Life at the End of Life: Finding Words Beyond Words* (Bristol, UK: Intellect, 2017), 16–17. See also Rita Charon, *Narrative Medicine: Honoring the Stories of Illness* (New York: Oxford University Press, 2006), and Rita Charon et al., *The Principles and Practice of Narrative Medicine* (New York: Oxford University Press, 2016).

9. In addition to *Life at the End of Life*, see my book *The Heart of the Hereafter: Love Stories from the End of Life* (Winchester, UK: Axis Mundi, 2014).

10. Regarding the value of adopting an integrated approach that combines the strengths of the liberal arts with STEM pedagogies, see the National Academies of Sciences, Engineering, and Medicine report, *The Integration of the Humanities and Arts with Sciences, Engineering, and Medicine in Higher Education: Branches of the Same Tree* (Washington, D.C.: The National Academies Press, 2018). Notably, I am not advocating that the humanities be placed in the service of applied disciplines. Instead, I am making a case for the power of collaborative interactions that can be beneficial for all involved.

11. It is a timely moment to be addressing these issues in medical communication. In 2016 Medicare began to provide reimbursement coverage for doctors to conduct end of life planning conversations with their patients. In part, this action came in response to a report issued by the Institute of Medicine of the National Academies, *Dying in America: Improving Quality and Honoring Individual Preferences Near the End of Life* (New York: National Academies Press, 2014). This report addresses not only the responsibilities of healthcare providers, but also of health system managers and policy makers in contributing to affordable, high-quality care at the end of life.

12. Lisa Howley, Elizabeth Gaufberg, and Brandy King, *The Fundamental Role of the Arts and Humanities in Medical Education* (Washington, D.C.: Association of American Medical Colleges, 2020), 1.

13. This observation relates not just to aesthetics, but also to related issues concerning how end of life insights are expressed and interpreted within a clinical setting, particularly when they engage subjects that exceed the familiar boundaries of language.

14. David Casarett, "Lessons in End-of-Life Care From the V.A.," *The New York Times* (November 11, 2015), http://opinionator.blogs.nytimes.com/2015/11/11/lessons-in-end-of-life-care-from-the-v-a/?action=click&pgtype=Homepage&clickSource=story-heading&module=opinion-c-col-right-region&region=opinion-c-col-right-region&WT.nav=opinion-c-col-right-region&_r=0.

15. Stein Kaasa et al., "Integration of Oncology and Palliative Care: A Lancet Oncology Commission," *Lancet Oncology* 19 (November 1, 2018), e588-e653, https://www.thelancet.com/journals/lanonc/article/PIIS1470-2045(18)30415-7/fulltext.

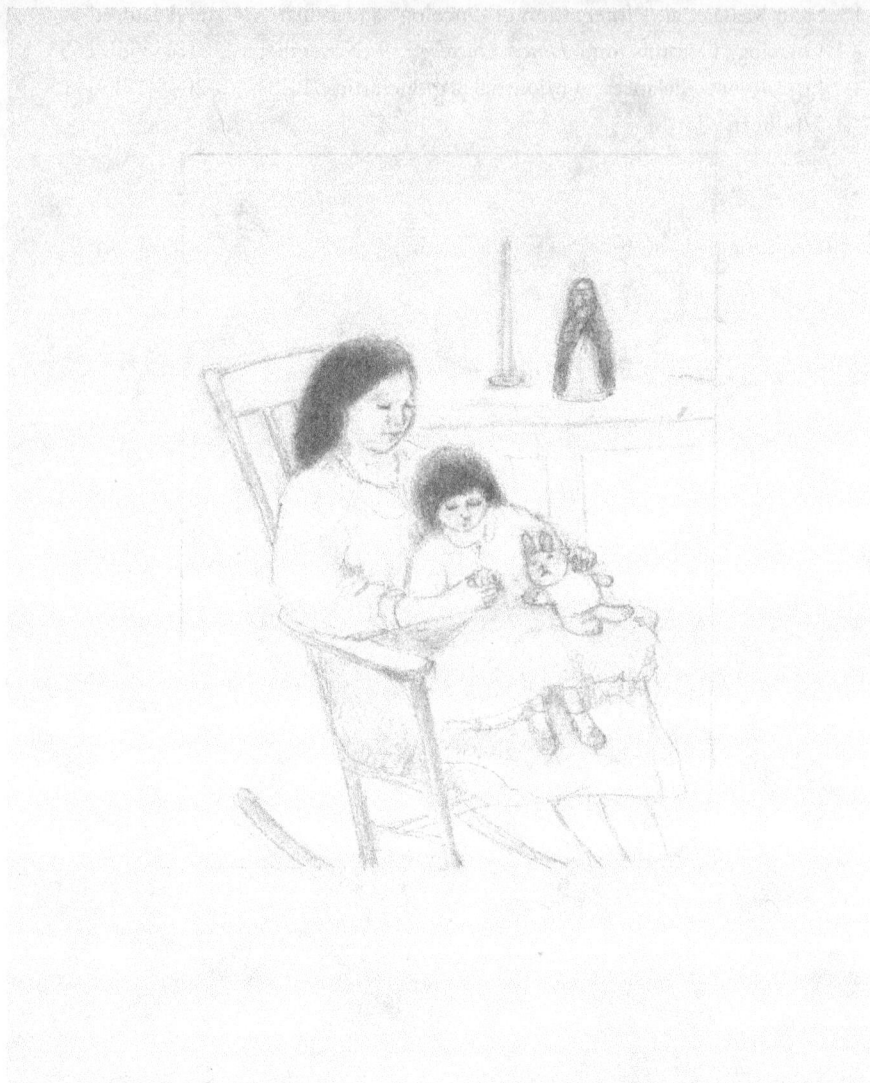

Figure 4: Lyn Smallwood, *Like Her Namesake*, 2016, graphite on white Arches paper

Chapter Two

A Rose From Two Gardens: Saint Thérèse of Lisieux and Images of the End of Life

Like Her Namesake: Having the Support of a Saint

"What a lovely little girl you have!"

"Thank you very much. Theresa, come over here and say hello."

Thus began my exchange with a young woman who had flown in earlier that morning so that she could be with her older brother who was passing away. Lying in the hospital bed, the man's breathing was slow and labored. As I listened to the distinctive gurgling sound that came from deep within his throat, I knew that he was actively dying.

When I first entered the Palliative Care Unit that day, other members of the medical team advised me that they found this family to be difficult to engage and closed off emotionally, as various family members took turns maintaining a vigil at the man's bedside. With these challenges in mind, I entered the room with no expectations whatsoever, just the desire to be present if the family wished to visit. After tapping gently on the door, I noticed a child playing in the far corner of the room, and I couldn't help but express my admiration for her. This proved to be a conversation opener. After chatting casually with the woman for a few minutes, I introduced myself and explained the work I do as an Artist In Residence. I then invited her to tell me something wonderful about her older brother. We had a lovely visit, producing a tribute to her brother that the other family members could contribute to, if they wished. When we had finished, we both looked over at the little girl who was quietly entertaining herself with a picture book and a stuffed animal. The woman then told me an extraordinary story about the birth of her daughter, whom she described as being

Like Her Namesake

My daughter is named for Saint Thérèse.
The doctors told me I was going to have a boy—
They even circled the gender on the ultrasound film.
The doctors also told me that
He could have some very serious health problems.

I was on my own at that time,
And I felt alone.
So, I looked around to find a saint to support me.
I came upon Saint Thérèse, and I said novenas to her.
I evoked her as my protector and patroness.

Then at nine months, my daughter was born.
She was a perfectly healthy girl,
And very beautiful.
Like her namesake.

When I first saw her,
I knew this was a sign,
And that Thérèse was on the job.
I knew that my prayers had been heard and answered.

God always hears these prayers.
They come from a place
Where everything is known.

In Lyn Smallwood's drawing (Figure 4), a young woman sits in a rocking chair, cradling a child in her lap. While the woman holds her daughter's hand, the little girl holds onto a small stuffed rabbit. Perched atop a cupboard are a devotional candle and a small statue of Saint Thérèse, whom the woman evoked for protection and grace as she prayed for the birth of a healthy child. The sweet faces of the mother and daughter bear a strong family resemblance. Both figures gaze downward at their two clasped hands, while nearby, Saint Thérèse appears to be watching over them. Such images speak to the importance of saints as protective presences and transitional figures, as well as to the instrumental ways in which people use symbolic objects to create a sense of

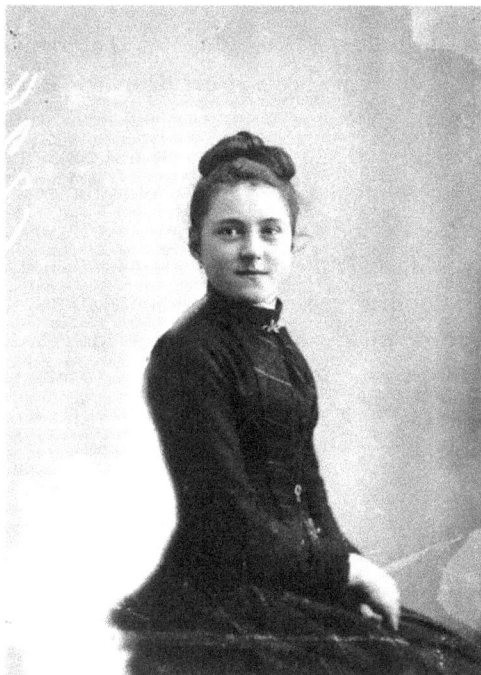

Figure 5: Mme. Besnier, Photograph
of Thérèse Martin, Lisieux, April
1888. Photo no. 4.
© Archives du Carmel de Lisieux,
http://www.archives-carmel-lisieux.fr/

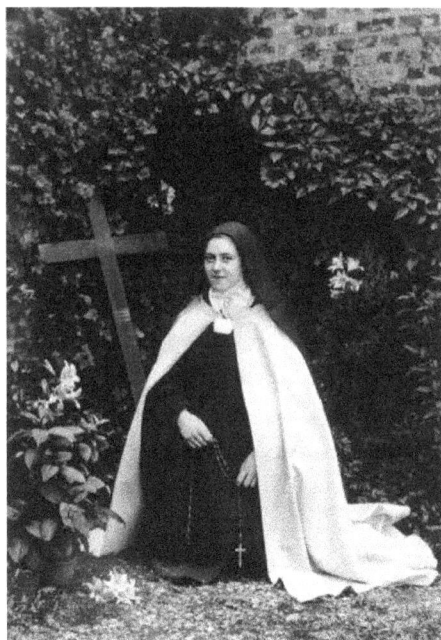

Figure 6: Céline Martin, Photograph of
Thérèse in the sacristy courtyard, July
1896. Photo no. 37. © Archives du
Carmel de Lisieux, http://www.archives-
carmel-lisieux.fr/

reciprocity between worlds and a common meeting place between them.

Before the birth of her daughter, and again, when facing the end of her brother's life, the woman turned to Saint Thérèse as a powerful source of strength and support, warmth and comfort. By engaging these existential and spiritual themes, this story evokes the convergence of multiple domains. Just as the narrative spans birth and death, it calls to mind the phases of life that unfold before the beginning and after the end of a discrete human lifespan. In the intimate setting of the hospital room, the woman described how her connection with Saint Thérèse provided her with a strong sense of accompaniment as she traversed these life passages. When viewed more broadly, this narrative also provides insight into how people envision the sacred in their lives, and how they see their own lives as sacred.

Who Is Thérèse? A Brief Account of the Life of Thérèse of Lisieux

This opening discussion raises a number of intriguing questions, perhaps the most immediate of which are: Who is Thérèse of Lisieux, and what is it about this particular saint that allows her to serve so broadly as a source of inspiration and accessibility? What supports the comparative parallel between this saintly life and the narratives of people facing the end of life? How do we account for the thematic similarities that arise within these very different cultural and historical contexts?

Thérèse Martin (Figures 5 and 6) was born on January 2, 1873 in Alençon, France, and she died of tuberculosis twenty-four years later at the Carmelite convent at Lisieux.[1] Thérèse was the youngest of five sisters, all of whom became nuns. Four of the Martin sisters joined the cloistered convent at Lisieux, while one sister joined the Visitation convent at Caen. Thérèse's mother, Marie-Azélie Guérin Martin, died when Thérèse was only four years old, leaving the older girls to serve as surrogate mothers. Thérèse entered the convent in April of 1888 at the age of fifteen. The previous year, Thérèse tried unsuccessfully to join the order. With her family, she traveled on a pilgrimage to Rome to celebrate the jubilee of Pope Leo XIII, the culmination of which was a public audience with the Pope, to whom Thérèse appealed directly for early entrance into the Carmel. Ultimately, Thérèse received her habit on January 10, 1889, and she professed her vows on September 8, 1890. From 1893 onward, Thérèse served as the convent's novice mistress, where she guided the spiritual formation of the newest members of the community. The

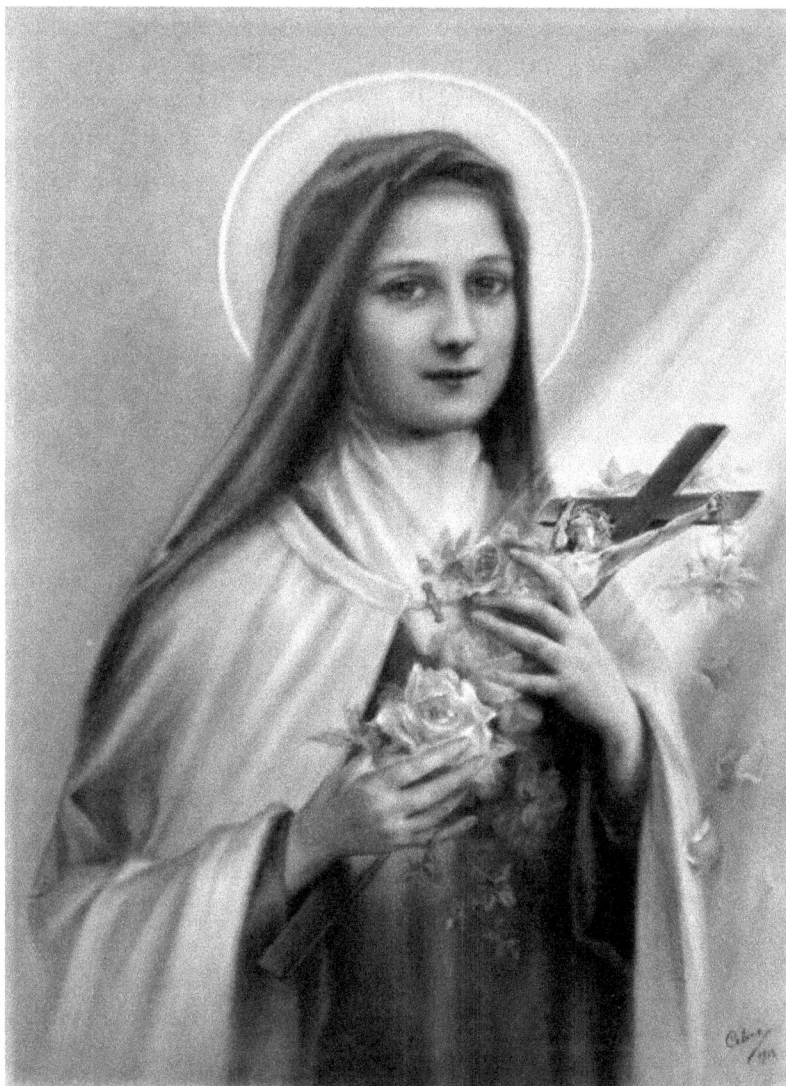

Figure 7: Céline Martin, Thérèse with Roses, 1912, charcoal. © Archives du Carmel de Lisieux, http://www.archives-carmel-lisieux.fr/

first indication of Thérèse's deadly illness appeared in the spring of 1896, as a hemorrhage of blood. For the next year and a half, Thérèse endured great pain and suffering. In the summer of 1897, she was moved to the convent infirmary, where she was personally attended by her sister Céline. Thérèse passed away on the evening of September 30, 1897.

At the request of her sister, in late 1894 Thérèse began to write the first section of her autobiography, which details the memories of her childhood and early life. Thérèse completed the initial portion of the text in early 1896. The briefer second and third sections were written in 1896 and 1897, respectively. The three sections were later assembled into a single volume under the title *Story of a Soul*. An edited version of the text was first published in 1898; an unedited version would not be released until 1956.[2] Shortly after its initial appearance, the book became a popular success. As the theologian Peter-Thomas Rohrbach has noted, Thérèse's autobiography

> ran through edition after edition. Between 1898 and 1915, over two hundred thousand copies of the French edition were published, and seven hundred thousand copies of the abridged French edition. By 1917, it had been translated into thirty-four languages or dialects. ... During the First World War, Thérèse became the darling of the troops in the French trenches. ... In Rome, Pope Benedict XV dispensed with the usual fifty-year waiting period, and allowed the investigations to be started for Thérèse's beatification.[3]

Rohrbach concludes that "The hurricane of glory reached its most intense peak in the 1920s. The miracles selected for her beatification and canonization were presented to the Congregation, and the clamor for that final honor continued throughout the Catholic world."[4] Thérèse was beatified in 1923, and she was officially canonized on May 17, 1925. Her feast day is October 1st. In October of 1997, Pope John Paul II named her a Doctor of the Church. On October 18, 2015 Thérèse's parents, Louis and Marie-Azélie Martin, were canonized by Pope Francis.

Just as Thérèse is associated with the autobiographical collection of writings assembled as *Story of a Soul*, statues of the saint currently serve as devotional images in churches and homes throughout the world. Indeed, Thérèse is one of the best known saints of our time. Lyn Smallwood's portrait, *That Rose Was Designated For Me* (Figure 1), is based on archival photographs of Thérèse that were taken by a commercial photographer in Lisieux in April of 1888 (Figure 5), and by her sister Céline in July of 1896 (Figure 6). Smallwood's drawing bears a closer resemblance to the historical likeness of Thérèse than many of the polychrome statues we encounter today, sculptures that tend to present the more slender facial features and the milder expression that are found in the famous charcoal drawing of *Thérèse with Roses* that Céline produced in 1912 (Figure 7).[5] Just as the subject of Smallwood's artwork is readily familiar, the softly nuanced qualities of the drawing make it feel evocative and visionary. By maintaining these complementary associations, the image can sustain a sense of clarity and ethereality, much like the character of Thérèse herself.

Why People Are Drawn to the Presences of Saints

While images of saints circulate widely in popular culture, saints are neither idols nor icons. That is, they are neither dazzling embodiments of a secular or pagan god who is displayed to be worshipped, nor are they splendid portals gesturing toward an infinite unknowable divinity. As the philosopher Jean-Luc Marion has observed, while the idol is a spectacle, the icon is an abyss.[6] Yet saints are neither spectacles nor abysses. Neither of these images conveys a human—or humanist—conception of the sacred. Instead, saints are human beings whose biographies offer existential reference points for accessing conceptions of the sacred within the framework of a human life. The figure of the saint thus continually negotiates the relations between humanity and divinity, while intrinsically shaping how the sacred can be seen and known in human terms. Just as saints mediate between these realms, they offer a vivid practical means to envision transformational presences. As one oncology patient told me:

> *I face a very daunting illness and a rough recovery.*
> *Yet I feel grateful for everything that's in my life.*
> *I'm a religious person.*
> *I believe strongly in God.*
> *I was raised Catholic,*
> *So I hold onto some of those ideals and descriptions.*
>
> *I feel like a lot of my prayers have been answered.*
> *I feel close to the saints, and to the Blessed Mother.*
> *I feel like they hear my prayers,*
> *And that strengthens my faith.*

Another day, I met a middle-aged woman whose husband was dying from throat cancer. As we produced a tribute honoring his life, the woman reflected on the importance of saints, and on how

We Don't Call On Them Enough

The older my husband has gotten,
The closer he's gotten to his faith.
He was in the construction business
And he is close to the carpenter, St. Joseph.
We also prayed to St. Blaise, for the throat.
And, I pray to Archangel Michael every day.
I believe in the power of saints and angels,
And we don't call on them enough.

In various ways, saints can serve as bridges between worlds. As an extremely accessible modern saint, Thérèse is associated with the "little way." In her writings Thérèse emphasized not the need to do great things, but the value of doing small things with great love. Combining seemingly oppositional conceptions of the great and the small, the "little way" represents an elegantly simple yet powerful spiritual practice that can seemingly be undertaken by everyone. For these reasons, the modernist painter Marsden Hartley once characterized Thérèse as an artist of the human soul whose life exemplified "precisely the office and the function of the mystic—to make the world aware that all these treasures are obtainable" by human beings.[7]

The Elevator and the Staircase: Images of Ascent and Descent

This sense of accessibility is one of the reasons why people often turn to Thérèse to feel a sense of connection and accompaniment when undertaking a challenging spiritual practice or when facing particularly difficult or painful life circumstances. Thérèse advocated adopting a simple and direct style of communication when seeking pathways of spiritual connection. This approach led to some of the images for which she is best known, namely, the staircase and the elevator. These images serve as both a practical and symbolic means for envisioning simultaneous pathways of ascent and descent.

When Thérèse first entered the Carmelite convent during the spring of 1888, she was assigned the lowly task of sweeping the staircase and dormitory.[8] The previous autumn, Thérèse and her family had traveled throughout Europe. In Paris, they visited the fashionable department store Le Printemps, where Thérèse encountered an elevator.[9] She later drew on these images as a means to envision bridging the gap between lofty spiritual aspirations and her self-conscious awareness of her human weakness and limitations.[10] To help overcome what she perceived as her own "littleness," Thérèse described her search for

> a means of going to heaven by a little way, a way that is very straight, very short, and totally new.

> We are living now in an age of inventions, and we no longer have to take the trouble of climbing stairs, for, in the homes of the rich, an elevator has replaced these very successfully. I wanted to find an elevator which would raise me to Jesus, for I am too small to climb the rough stairway of perfection.[11]

As Thérèse searched the scriptures for insight on how to accomplish this goal, she recognized that "The elevator which must raise me to heaven is Your arms, O Jesus! And for this I had no need to grow up, but rather I had to remain *little* and become this more and more."[12] The staircase and the elevator thus enabled Thérèse to clothe elevated spiritual images in very practical, tangible, and accessible forms. Thérèse's great humility, coupled with her knowledge of a modern technological device, provided an effective means to imagine a pathway of spiritual ascent through uplift in the arms of divine presence.[13]

Uplift: The Stairway with Columns

In both Thérèse's writings and in contemporary end-of-life narratives, the image of an ascending pathway can provide a vivid metaphor to imagine practical routes leading to transcendent planes. One day I met an older woman who lay propped up in bed, at the very end of her life, surrounded by her adult children. When I first entered the room, two of the woman's daughters were in the room, and another daughter and a son arrived a little later. As the woman and I began to visit, she sent her family out of the room so that she could speak freely, without inhibition or interruption. Once the narrative was complete, she invited everyone back in to hear her evocative story:

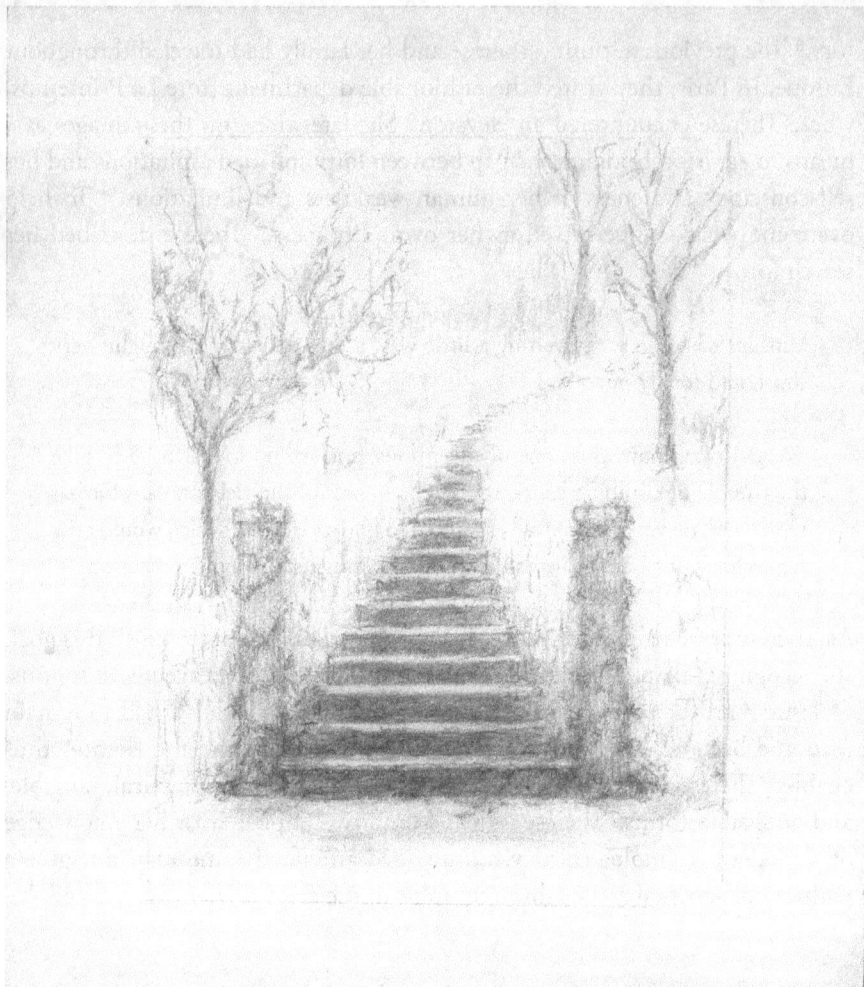

Figure 8: Lyn Smallwood, *Uplift: The Stairway with Columns*, 2015, graphite on white Arches paper

Uplift: The Stairway with Columns

For my image,
There's a favorite portrait of a stairway
That I like to glance at, at home.
It's a stairway with columns and leaves and ivies.
It's pinkish and greenish, and it's in a gold frame.
It's been in my bedroom for many years.
It was a gift to me.
I like the color schemes, and the two pretty pillars.
I like to think that it's leading up to heaven,
Or, onto a path that is beautiful.
It's almost like a stairway going up.
It just leads up—
I don't want to say to the clouds—
It just kind of fades at the top.

It makes me feel good to know that there is such a beautiful place.
It makes me think of security, peace, no pain, and happy people.
It makes me think about what I've always wondered about,
To bring happiness into my life.

To me, it has a special meaning,
Not only because it is beautiful,
But because it just does.
This image does have a sparkle,
In the pinkish light,
And a sense of uplift.

It's a sacred image.
I've asked myself, "What could I find that would actually match it?"
Nothing comes close to it.
It's a beauty that I don't like anyone to touch.
It's a beauty that lies between me, the moment, and the picture.

While facing the end of her life, the woman reflected on how the image of the staircase evoked a place of peace, beauty, and comfort. The visionary aesthetics of this idyllic scene inspired thoughts of the sacred, as the woman contemplated the transitional space that lay "between me, the moment, and the picture." Lyn Smallwood's drawing *Uplift: The Stairway with Columns* (Figure 8) was inspired by the description of a winding stone staircase flanked by two fluted marble columns. Vines of ivy twist gracefully around the classical pillars that mark the entrance to the scene, while a gently curving stairway leads upward, ultimately fading at the top of the drawing. Much like Thérèse's images, this artwork presents a scene that is at once practical and metaphysical, naturalistic and transcendent. The drawing's emphatic pencil lines are densely clustered along the base of the image, evoking a solid surface at the contact point where the stairs and the columns connect to the earth. The image then becomes increasingly abstract as the scene winds gently upward through a delicate landscape filled with trees and grasses, and it ultimately vanishes as it leads to a point beyond what can be seen.

The Circular Porch: Going All the Way Around

The writings of Thérèse of Lisieux and of people at the end of life often evoke passageways spanning multiple worlds. One day I met an older man who suffered from an extremely aggressive form of renal cell carcinoma. The man expressed a deep sense of sadness and fear, as he had already lost several relatives to this illness. As we visited, I asked the man about the images that were meaningful for him. While I remained deeply attuned to his experiences of pain and suffering, as he spoke, I was also listening closely for the transformational elements to emerge. Ultimately, these themes appeared through a striking image of struggle and ascension, just as his story came full circle to reach an elevated, transitional space:

> *The Circular Porch: Going All the Way Around*
>
> *My image now would be to die in a peaceful manner.*
> *That is the opposite of where I seem to be headed.*
> *When you're a kid, you're naïve.*
> *There is a lot that is never spoken about.*
> *There's a lot of cancer in my family.*
> *As you get older, you become more aware of things.*
>
> *I am from Iowa, originally, and I remember Sunday afternoons,*
> *Getting into the family car and driving up to the hills.*
> *These were rough mud roads, and we'd have to get out and push the car.*

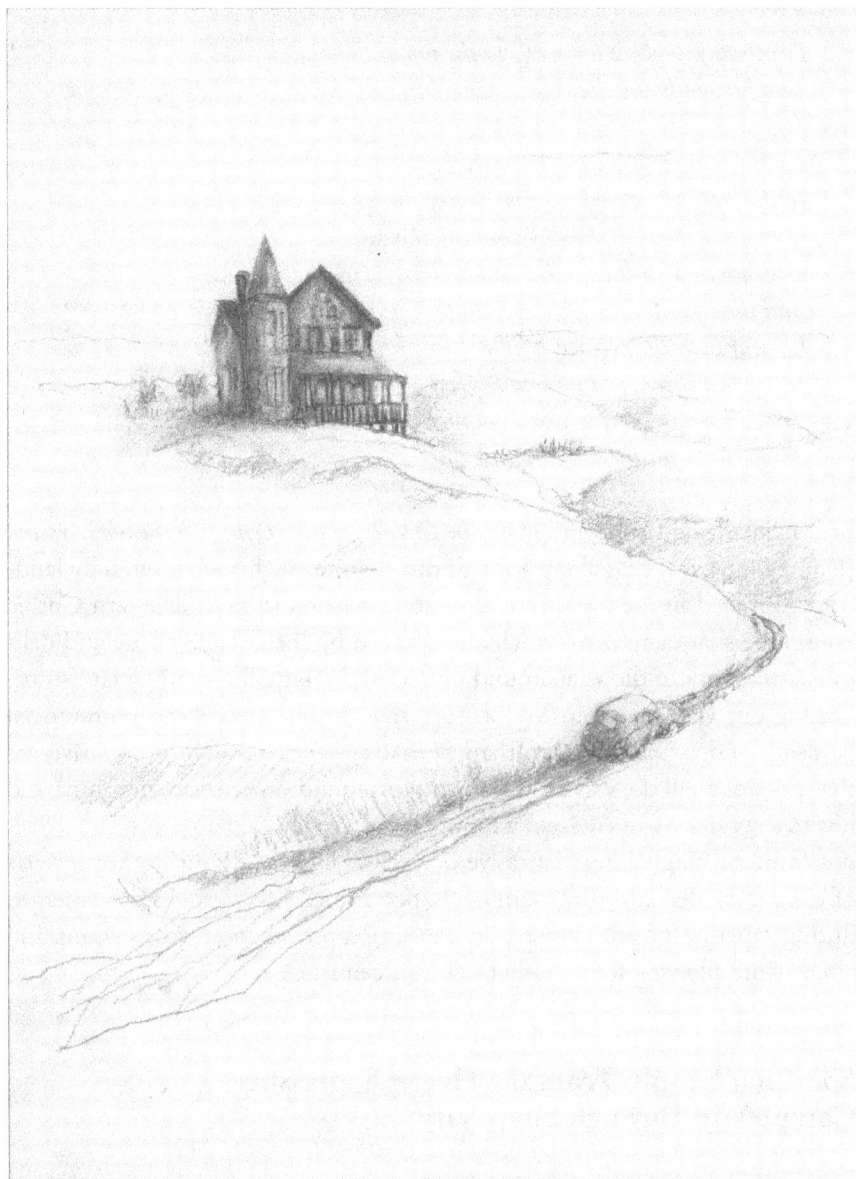

Figure 9: Lyn Smallwood, *The Circular Porch: Going All the Way Around*, 2020, graphite on white Strathmore drawing paper

Eventually we'd get up there, to the top of the hill,
To a big old house that had a big white porch going all the way around.

I'm thinking of this now because,
In life, you go through all these crazy things,
Like going through the day, pushing the car,
Getting stuck in the mud, and laughing, and getting mad.
And then you finally get there, and it's just a different world.
It's your own little world, and nothing affects you badly.
You're just there, and it's totally good.
You can see a different world up there, from the circular porch,
As you walk all the way around.

In Lyn Smallwood's illustration of *The Circular Porch: Going All the Way Around* (Figure 9), a car travels along a rough dirt road through a winding, hilly landscape. Perched in the distance is the silhouette of a large Midwestern Gothic house, the sharp angles of which are softened by the circular sweep and delicate latticework of the wraparound porch overlooking the winding landscape. During our visit, the man told a story that encompassed both pronounced hardship and striking beauty, themes that emerged through a narrative arc that extended "all the way around," from profound experiences of trauma and loss to the capacity to envision a more expansive view. Notably, this story does not feature a single linear narrative of decline into death, but rather, a sense of circularity that overturns familiar expectations. Just as this story emerged during a period of pronounced darkness, it expresses a sense of coming full circle while allowing for a moment of transcendence.

Speaking Simply, From the Heart: Expressing Complexity Through Simplicity

When I work with people at the end of life, their statements seem both familiar and poetic, as they repeatedly draw on their concrete life experiences to express subtle states of being. Throughout *Story of a Soul*, Thérèse similarly advocated taking a simple and direct approach to life and language. As a Discalced Carmelite nun, Thérèse was often in a state of prayer, and her writings are filled with allusions to sacred texts. Yet instead of selecting formal prayers from prayer books, Thérèse advocated adopting familiar speech patterns in prayer, which sometimes led her to joyful and expansive spiritual states. As she wrote:

"I say very simply to God what I wish to say, without composing beautiful sentences, and He always understands me. For me, *prayer* is an aspiration of the heart, it is a simple glance directed to heaven, it is a cry of gratitude and love in the midst of trial as well as joy; finally, it is something great, supernatural, which expands my soul…"[14]

The keynote of Thérèse's approach is her sense of simplicity and sincerity. Implicit in her words is the very powerful insight that language has a life all its own. When people speak of matters that are close to the heart, their language cannot be forced or contrived. Familiar speech patterns create space for individuals to speak openly and to recognize the power of their own words. I have found that when engaging both Thérèse's writings and the stories people tell at the end of life, clear and simple statements often convey profound depths of insight. When I was presenting this work to a group of dental students, a third-year student observed that the narratives are important "because you see your patients as human beings. It is so important to have this simple, authentic language expressed in poetic form. Typically, poetry is seen as a high art form that is not for everyone." The stories in this book exemplify the ways in which *everyone* has the potential for such creative expression.

Both Ordinary and Extraordinary: Visionary Traditions and Vernacular Mysticism

Beyond their shared emphasis on the familiar dynamics of inclusive presence, how do we account for the parallels between Thérèse's writings and the stories people tell at the end of life? Thérèse was raised in a devoutly religious family, and her brief adult life unfolded in a cloistered Carmelite convent. Within these sheltered conditions, Thérèse was an extraordinary person who lived in the ordinary circumstances of her time. Similarly, individuals at the end of life are ordinary people living in extraordinary—yet universally human—conditions. Both Thérèse and people at the end of life know firsthand the painful and debilitating effects of deadly illnesses. They constantly confront situations that require them to consider the ways in which life can extend beyond the boundaries of the physical body, and how transcendent subjects can be experienced and expressed in human terms. The comparison of Thérèse and people facing the end of life thus invites us to consider the ways in which extremely restricted life situations, which are marked by a sense of finite boundaries and limited mobility, can help to create the conditions for intense reflection and heightened states of consciousness. Facing the end of life—or its imminent possibility—can be an experience so radical that it confirms certain aspects of the self, just as it takes the person beyond familiar conceptions of the self. Paradoxically, the experience can simultaneously affirm and destabilize an individual's identity while creating the possibility for expansive visions to emerge.[15]

Just as she lived an ordinary human life, Thérèse's mystical life encompassed the prophetic, noetic, and clairsentient domains. As discussed in Chapter Seven, Thérèse linked the themes of knowledge and ineffability to extreme states of light and darkness, thereby describing a state of being that could encompass nondual aspects of vision and blindness. While her writings clearly belong to a visionary tradition, Thérèse's spiritual images are repeatedly clothed in language that is intimate, familiar, and vernacular.

Thérèse's mystical gifts became evident during early childhood. At the age of six, she expressed advance knowledge of a family tragedy as she received a clairvoyant image that foreshadowed her father's devastating neurological illness many years later. Following her own profoundly disturbing experience with a prolonged childhood illness, Thérèse described a transformative healing encounter in which a statue of the Virgin Mary as *Our Lady of Victories* became alive and smiled at her (Figure 10). In the *Novissima Verba*—the compilation of last words that her sisters recorded at the end of her life—Thérèse described various telepathic incidents and synchronistic events. These included her desiring, and subsequently receiving, a particular item, and of sending certain thoughts remotely to her sister Céline, who then communicated these ideas to Thérèse during a subsequent visit.[16] Thérèse also expressed precognitive knowledge of her own early death, and she correctly predicted that she would become a great saint.

Yet Thérèse was also a very humble and practical person. She did not seek ecstatic experiences of mystical union which, as the historian Thomas R. Nevin has noted, were considered to be suspect as they were associated with conceptions of medieval "illuminism."[17] When facing the end of her life, Thérèse candidly told one of her fellow nuns that "I can nourish myself on nothing but the truth. This is why I've never wanted any visions. We can't see, here on earth, heaven, the angels, etc., just as they are. I prefer to wait until after my death."[18] Yet Thérèse admitted to having one such ecstatic experience, which occurred shortly after she made her Act of Oblation. When asked to describe her mystical experience, Thérèse recounted how

> suddenly, I was seized with such a violent love for God that I can't explain it except by saying it felt as though I were totally plunged into fire. Oh! What fire and what sweetness at one and the same time! I was on fire with

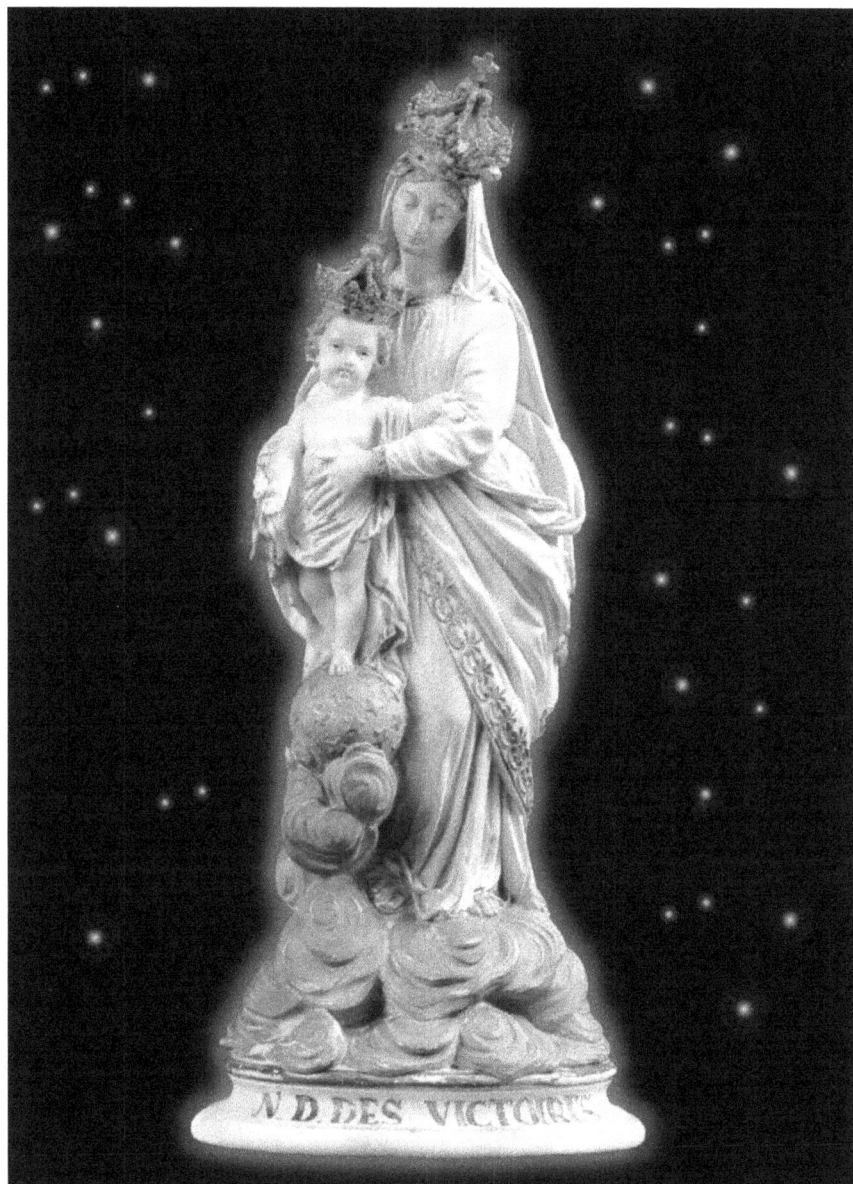

Figure 10: Statue of Our Lady of Victories, kept in the Infirmary of the Convent at the Carmel of Lisieux. © Archives du Carmel de Lisieux, http://www.archives-carmel-lisieux.fr/

love, and I felt that one minute more, one second more, and I wouldn't be able to sustain this ardor without dying. I understood, then, what the saints were saying about these states which they experienced so often. As for me, I experienced it only once and for one single instant.[19]

Thérèse's emphasis on the brevity and modesty of her experience is consistent with her overall sense of humility and simplicity. Throughout her writings, Thérèse expressed an acute awareness of her own "littleness" and the joy she felt in merging with a power far greater than herself. In *Story of a Soul* she also expressed these subjects paradoxically, by *not* describing them. She recalled that, during her First Communion, she experienced a profound love and a sense of "fusion; there were no longer two, Thérèse had vanished as a drop of water is lost in the immensity of the ocean." She then declined to comment further, noting, "I don't want to enter into detail here. There are certain things that lose their perfume as soon as they are exposed to the air; there are deep *spiritual thoughts* which cannot be expressed in human language without losing their intimate and heavenly meaning."[20]

But He Knew: Knowing the Unknowable

Like Thérèse, people at the end of life will sometimes recall vivid, powerful dreams in which they experience being in multiple locations at once and visiting with spiritual presences. These subjects are discussed in Chapter Eight. Dying people will also sometimes express clairvoyant knowledge of otherwise unknowable events. One day, I visited with a middle-aged man whose young son lay in bed, facing the end of life from an aggressive form of pancreatic cancer. A few days earlier, the young man was still able to speak, and various family members took turns staying overnight at the hospital. As I visited with the father, he described an extraordinary event that had occurred two nights before:

But He Knew

My son woke up at 4 a.m. and he said,
"Dad, someone is stealing from us."
We called the house, and the family did a quick inventory.
Everything was fine.
There was no one in the house, and nothing was missing.

Then yesterday, we found out
That someone had gotten into one of the credit card accounts,
And they had stolen several thousand dollars' worth of merchandise.
Through intuition,
My son knew it was happening.
He couldn't pinpoint it.
But, he knew.

Such stories are both simple and powerful. Expressed in straightforward language, the narratives describe events that are both ordinary and extraordinary.

Sugar and Vinegar: The Intimacy and the Distance of Saints and People at the End of Life

In the bull of canonization of 1925, Pope Pius XI noted that Thérèse of Lisieux achieved sanctity "without going beyond the common order of things."[21] This papal pronouncement sheds further light on the comparison between Thérèse and people at the end of life, as well as the saint's status as both an appealing *and* a particularly challenging figure. As the theologian Mary Frohlich has observed, "In every corner of the globe, one will find some form of shrine to St. Thérèse in many Roman Catholic churches. A recent world-wide tour of her relics drew crowds in the tens of thousands at nearly every stop." Frohlich associates Thérèse's popularity with her gift for encouraging others to identify with her example. Thus Thérèse "places herself as an equal in the midst of the masses of simple folk who will never be specially noticed or acclaimed. In so doing, she affirms and embraces the capability of each one to follow her in her 'little way' of sanctity."[22]

Just as Thérèse is so widely seen and honored, so too has she "sometimes been dismissed, especially by people of higher levels of education and sophistication, on the grounds that her protected and childlike life had little in common with their own."[23] Regarding this issue, Thomas R. Nevin has observed that, while some devout people are put off by Thérèse's seeming perfection, others have expressed disdain for the ordinariness of her example:

It would not be amiss to claim that [Thérèse] is the most beloved woman in modern history, certainly among Catholics. But she is both too easily embraced and too easily dismissed: a saint of common people, presumably, accessible to everyone. ... She is one of us and, being so, she says that sainthood is for anybody. So say her devotees. And, by the same turn, she is some-times dismissed as a simpering, if not simple-minded, creature, a mediocrity in intellect.[24]

These statements reveal a suggestive paradox, as Thérèse is critiqued for being both too high and too low, for exemplifying unattainable perfection and for her seemingly banal associations with bourgeois sentimentality.[25] In her life-time, Thérèse characterized the praise and the scorn that she received from oth-ers as expressions of sugar and vinegar, and in her humility, she expressed her preference for the latter.[26] Through the opposite yet complementary images of sugar and vinegar, Thérèse found a vivid metaphor to frame contrasting associations while investing ordinary life with heightened spiritual meanings. By coupling the distinctive imagery of sugar and vinegar, Thérèse presented an intriguing metaphor, not only for encouragement and disparagement, but for the ambivalent sense of attraction and repulsion that I have repeatedly witnessed between the living and the dying.

For individuals such as saints who are human beings living extraordinary lives—and for ordinary people facing the extraordinary terrain of the end of life—the far edges of the existential spectrum can become pronounced. Both their suffering and their exaltation can seem unreal and otherworldly. Given these extreme states of being, people often both can and can't identify with saints and with people at the end of life, as their presences can seem too real *and* too visionary.

In turn, the writings of saints and of people at the end of life can be seen as both a regressive and a transgressive genre, a corpus that variously risks romanticizing death while over-privileging conceptions of spirituality. In both cases, the texts engage the subjectivity of suffering human beings who present ready targets for being critiqued, pathologized, or otherwise managed. As the scholars Françoise Meltzer and Jaś Elsner have noted, when engaging with holy figures such as saints, "When excess is named, the act of naming itself either domesticates its radicality or appropriates it into an ideological discourse susceptible to dismissal and manipulation."[27] They further observe that saintly excess is associated with conceptions of grace, miracles, surrender, mystery, charisma, joy, and the real. My experiences have repeatedly shown me that something similar occurs at the end of life, a transitional time when individuals may be associated with extraordinary conceptions of power and authority, just as they are also subject to intense objectification, vulnerability, and dismissal. In both cases, these lives can be dissociated from the familiar conditions of life itself, particularly as people appear to be repellant or attractive, banal or sacred—and sometimes, both at once.

Indeed, due to their exceptional life circumstances, both saints and people at the end of life can be readily embraced or dismissed as outliers within normative human life. Conjoining the ordinary and the extraordinary, such lives are positioned at the very edges of human experience. For these reasons, both can be associated with domains that are too high and too low, while engendering polarizing conceptions of the superhuman and the subhuman—associations that can be dissociated from shared conceptions of our common humanity. When end-of-life experience becomes predominantly associated with personal disintegration and suffering, people tend to become objectified and lose their sense of humanity, and people may turn away in fear and repulsion.[28] In turn, when human life becomes overly rarified or sanctified, a person can seem otherworldly and excessively idealized. In either case, by becoming unreachable and untouchable, the person becomes less real to others around them. In my experience, the key is to cultivate strategies for spanning the distance between these states of being and finding ways to bridge the gap between them.

I Fold Again, Into the Memory: Bridging Multiple Worlds

I will close with a story that exemplifies what it can mean to live in multiple locations at once, to reach a place where ascent and descent become interwoven within a single inclusive gesture. One day I worked with two older Catholic priests who were Missionaries of Our Lady of La Salette. Their order is named for a small town in the French Alps where, in September of 1846, an apparition of a beautiful lady, who was later identified as the Blessed Virgin, appeared to two shepherd children. In 1852, the religious order was founded to honor the vision and the message of reverence and healing that this holy figure imparted.

One of the priests imminently faced the end of his life, while his dear friend and colleague of many years sat attentively at his bedside. While the man at the end of life became extremely anxious when medical matters were being discussed, he was remarkably calm and lucid when recounting subjects close to his heart. As the three of us sat together reflecting on the men's life experiences and the images that were significant for them, the two priests spoke movingly about their order's place of origin in France. As the men reminisced about the profundity of their experiences there, their voices blended to form a composite narrative:

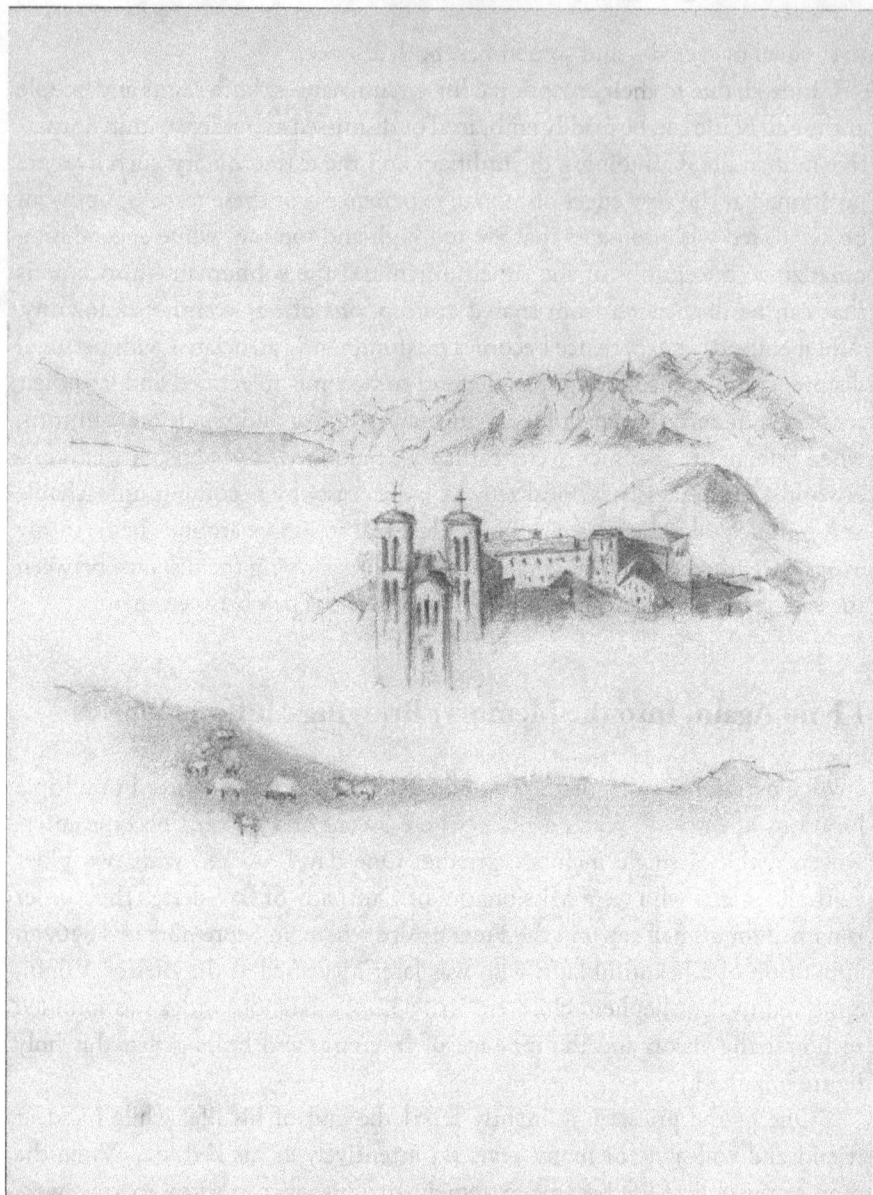

Figure 11: Lyn Smallwood, *I Fold Again, Into the Memory*, 2020, graphite on white Strathmore drawing paper

I Fold Again, Into the Memory

We are Missionaries of Our Lady of La Salette.
We both worked in the French Alps, at La Salette.
It all began there—it's the site of the vision.
That's what brought us together:
The Alps and the Shrine.
It's 6,000 feet up, so it's at a high elevation.
It's like, there are peaks all around.
There's a church there,
And when you get up in the morning,
You are in a sea of clouds.
At about 10 in the morning the clouds just lift,
And it's incredible.
In the summer there are sheep and goats,
And you can hear the bells around their necks.
It's a quiet place,
A prayerful place.

This sense of prayerfulness also came this morning,
As I was holding my friend's hand
And we were praying the Our Father together.
We were in a prayerful place.
We were all there for one purpose:
Unity.

When you're there, in that place,
It's difficult to imagine that all of this is really happening.
So now,
I fold again,
Into the memory.

Lyn Smallwood's illustration (Figure 11) presents an evocative view of this visionary landscape. In the drawing's foreground, sheep graze gently on an Alpine hillside, while at a distance, we see the dramatic architecture of the church and the shrine encircled by mountain peaks. Through the juxtaposition of solids and voids, the church appears to be poised in an etheric field of clouds, an effect that is created using the negative space of the drawing. As the men told a story of prayer and unity set within this strikingly beautiful natural setting, their narrative evoked a complementary sense of a parallel reality that is simultaneously real and mystical, pastoral and visionary, grounded and transcendent.

Like many of the artworks that appear in this book, *I Fold Again, Into the Memory* fuses seemingly oppositional states of being into a unified sense of presence. This story expresses a nondual sense of the high and the low, intimacy and distance, supplication and devotion, humility and empowerment. As we visited together, the men shared a narrative that went deep and high. As the priests bow and fold, so too do they rise and lift. Through such apparently ordinary motions, the men move in two seemingly opposite directions at once as they reach a place of oneness. During our visit, this singular act of doubling appeared in a story that evoked a landscape of life and death. As I sat there listening to their story, I knew that I was in the presence of a rose from two gardens.

Notes

1. The bibliography on Thérèse of Lisieux is extensive. The sources that primarily inform my discussion include Thérèse de Lisieux, *Story of a Soul: The Autobiography of Saint Thérèse of Lisieux*, 3rd ed., trans. John Clarke (Washington, D.C.: ICS Publications, 1996); Thérèse de Lisieux, *St. Thérèse of Lisieux: Her Last Conversations*, trans. John Clarke (Washington, D.C.: ICS Publications, 1977); Thomas R. Nevin, *Thérèse of Lisieux: God's Gentle Warrior* (New York: Oxford University Press, 2006); Thomas R. Nevin, *The Last Years of Saint Thérèse: Doubt and Darkness, 1895–1897* (New York: Oxford University Press, 2013); and Peter-Thomas Rohrbach, *The Search for Saint Thérèse* (Garden City, NY: Doubleday, 1961). Additional sources include Herbert J. Thurston and Donald Attwater's discussion of "St. Teresa of Lisieux" in *Butler's Lives of the Saints*, vol. 4 (Westminster, MD: Christian Classics, 1990), 12–16; and the entries on the saint found in David Hugh Farmer, *The Oxford Dictionary of Saints*, 2nd ed. (New York: Oxford University Press, 1987), 405-6; Donald Attwater, ed., *A Dictionary of Saints* (London: Burns & Oates, 1958), 251; and Richard P. McBrien, *The HarperCollins Encyclopedia of Catholicism* (San Francisco: HarperSanFrancisco, 1995), 1251–52.
2. For a detailed history of the evolution of the individual texts that were later assembled as *Story of a Soul*, including the ordering of the manuscripts, significant editorial changes, and relevant discussions concerning Thérèse's original addressees and readers, see Nevin, *The Last Years of Saint Thérèse*, 164–74.
3. Rohrbach, *The Search for St. Thérèse*, 218–19.
4. Rohrbach, *The Search for St. Thérèse*, 223.
5. Céline's original charcoal drawing, and the historical photographs of Thérèse that appear in this chapter, are housed in the Archives of the Carmel at Lisieux and they are reproduced with the convent's permission. For Céline's discussion of the work that the charcoal portrait was meant to accomplish as an image within mass circulation, see the artist's notes on this piece at http://archives-carmel-lisieux.fr/english/carmel/index.php/autres/867-st-therese-with-roses-1912-charcoal-by-celine.
6. Jean-Luc Marion, *God Without Being: Hors-Texte*, 2nd ed., trans. Thomas A. Carlson (1991; Chicago: University of Chicago Press, 2012), Chapter One.
7. Marsden Hartley, "St. Thérèse of Lisieux," *On Art by Marsden Hartley*, ed. Gail R. Scott (New York: Horizon Press, 1982), 161.

8. Thérèse recounts performing these tasks in *St. Thérèse of Lisieux*, 95, 107.

9. As discussed in Nevin, *Thérèse of Lisieux*, 50.

10. As Nevin has pointed out, when Thérèse described the elevator imagery during the summer of 1897, she was well aware of her grave physical illness and her impending death, having become "so debilitated by fever and lack of nutrition, being unable to digest most of what was given her … she could barely climb the stairs to her room." See Nevin, *Thérèse of Lisieux*, 201.

11. Quoted in *Story of a Soul*, 207. Regarding this imagery, see also p. 49 of this volume.

12. Quoted in *Story of a Soul*, 208.

13. Thérèse drew on related imagery of spiritual uplift and attainment when talking with her sister Céline. In a moment of anticipatory grief, Céline recalled asking, "Do you believe I can still hope to be with you in heaven? This seems impossible to me. It's like expecting a cripple with one arm to climb to the top of a greased pole to fetch an object." To which Thérèse replied, "Yes, but if there's a giant there who picks up the little cripple in his arms, raises him high, and gives him the object desired! This is exactly what God will do for you." Quoted in *St. Thérèse of Lisieux*, 221.

14. Quoted in *Story of a Soul*, 242.

15. Facing the end of life can engender a sense of what the philosopher Jean-Luc Marion has, in another context, termed the self beyond the self, which represents a creative means of re-envisioning oneself, other people, the world, and divinity. Regarding this formulation, see Jean-Luc Marion, *In the Self's Place: The Approach of Saint Augustine*, trans. Jeffrey L. Kosky (Chicago: University of Chicago Press, 2012).

16. These telepathic and synchronistic incidents are recounted in *St. Thérèse of Lisieux*, 168, 93.

17. Nevin, *Thérèse of Lisieux*, ix, 116, 158.

18. Quoted in *St. Thérèse of Lisieux*, 134.

19. Quoted in *St. Thérèse of Lisieux*, 77.

20. Quoted in *Story of a Soul*, 77.

21. As quoted in Peter-Thomas Rohrbach, "Thérèse of Lisieux," *Encyclopedia of Religion*, 2nd ed., vol. 13, ed. Lindsay Jones (Detroit: Macmillan Reference, 2005), 9155.

22. Mary Frohlich, *St. Thérèse of Lisieux: Essential Writings* (Maryknoll, NY: Orbis Books, 2007), 13–14.

23. Frohlich, *St. Thérèse of Lisieux*, 15.

24. Nevin, *Thérèse of Lisieux*, ix. These issues also emerge in the historical bibliography on Thérèse. Vita Sackville-West approaches related questions through a

critical comparison of Thérèse of Lisieux and Teresa of Avila in *The Eagle and the Dove* (1943; London: Pan Macmillan, 2011). For a psychoanalytically inflected reading of Thérèse's life, see Monica Furlong, *Thérèse of Lisieux* (London: Virago, 1987). One of the most historically influential psychoanalytical readings of Thérèse is found in Etienne Robo, *Two Portraits of St. Teresa of Lisieux* (Glasgow: Sands, 1955). In *The Hidden Face: A Study of St. Thérèse of Lisieux* (Freiburg im Breisgau: Herder Verlag, 1959), Ida Görres asserts that Thérèse's example negatively engenders a sense of inferiority and littleness in others. For an account of this early historiography, and for a response to Thérèse's critics who variously expressed charges of fraud, sentimental pietism, and neurosis, see Rohrbach, *The Search for St. Thérèse*.

25. As Nevin succinctly observes, the complex question of whether Thérèse can provide "a model for the conjunction of revelation and human personality in situ" represents a concern of fundamental theology. See Nevin, *Thérèse of Lisieux*, 317.

26. Quoted in *Story of a Soul*, 244.

27. Françoise Meltzer and Jaś Elsner, "Introduction," *Saints: Faith Without Borders*, ed. Françoise Meltzer and Jaś Elsner (Chicago: University of Chicago Press, 2011), ix, x. As Meltzer and Elsner note, while the modern scientific world has dismissed the saint as a kind of primitive throwback, this figure reflects a postmodern fascination with states of excess, marginality, porousness, and transgression. By providing a way to think outside of normative social patterns, the holy person thus represents "a queer[ing of] stable binary structures" while enacting "vertical" access to supernatural realms and divine power. As such, saints are figures who remain magical, uncomfortable, non-normative, and excessive.

28. For a critical account of the ways in which an individual's identity becomes eroded in the dying process as the body falls into states of decay, see Julia Lawton's classic account of "dirty dying" in *The Dying Process: Patients' Experiences of Palliative Care* (New York: Routledge, 2000).

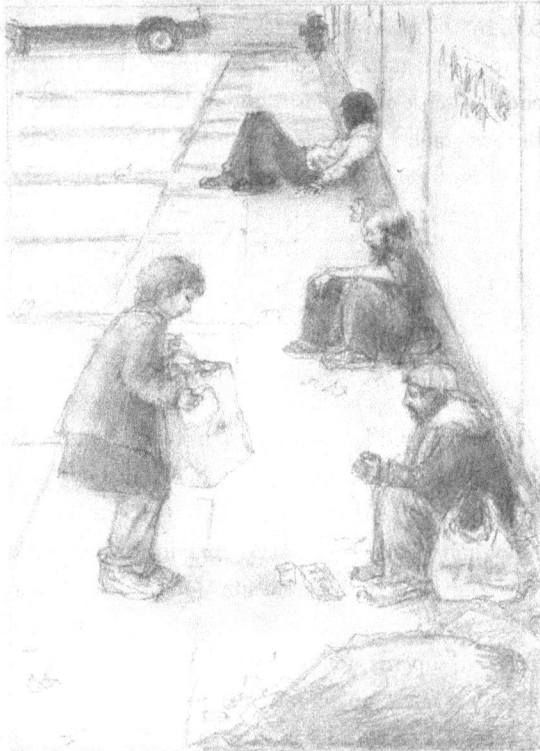

Figure 12: Lyn Smallwood, *Feeding the Homeless: The Capacity to Love*, 2015, graphite on white Arches paper

Chapter Three

The Grandeur of the Smallest Things: Charity, Caregiving, and the "Little Way"

Feeding the Homeless: Humility and the Capacity to Love

The woman in the bed was actively dying, and she was barely able to move or speak. As I visited with her family, I learned that the woman had dedicated a substantial portion of her life to performing charitable activities and engaging in social service work. Standing at the bedside, we went around in a circle and people told a remarkable story about the woman's compassionate character, and how she put her ideals into action. The woman's younger sister proudly recalled how, for many years, the two had ventured out onto the city streets at night in order to undertake activities close to their hearts:

Feeding the Homeless: The Capacity to Love

My sister has a beautiful heart,
And a beautiful spirit.
She loved to go and feed the homeless.
We would put the food and the drinks in the car,
And go right out there,
On the streets of the city.
She never had any trouble.
Not once.

She put herself out there,
With compassion
And the capacity to love.

She and I would do this,
And we did it for years.

We did it because of the need,
And it made us feel wonderful.

Lyn Smallwood's drawing, *Feeding the Homeless: The Capacity to Love* (Figure 12), displays an urban scene at dusk. On the downtown streets of a big city, an unassuming middle-aged woman walks quietly along the edge of the pavement, carrying a bulky tote bag filled with food. As she passes by, she distributes sandwiches to the row of men who sit huddled on the concrete sidewalk, their backs pressed against the graffiti-covered wall. The rounded contours of the men's vulnerable forms contrast with the sharp geometry of the hard sidewalk. In the immediate foreground we see the woman approaching a crouching man. Wearing an old jacket and a dirty cap, the man squats on the sidewalk among incidental pieces of trash while he extends a hand outward to receive the woman's offering. Additional men appear in a long row along the edge of the city block. Their punctuated figures draw the viewer's gaze back into the scene, toward the people whom the woman will soon approach. Both the drawing and the narrative convey a sense of walking into an unknown world. Just as viewers encounter a scene that is deeply rooted in hard reality, the imagery reflects the tenderness of serving the underserved, of entering a place where small things can mean almost everything.

Such acts of charity appear as leitmotifs in end-of-life narratives and in the writings of Thérèse of Lisieux. The stories repeatedly emphasize the ways in which seemingly small gestures can hold worlds of meaning and value. While pursuing a spiritual practice that she called the "little way," Thérèse explored how the sacred could be perceived in such modest acts of care—particularly in gestures that involved the grace of self-overcoming, in which an individual placed the needs of others before themselves.[1] In end-of-life narratives, these activities range from apparently incidental gestures of compassion to larger philanthropic acts in which a person provides support and comfort to those in need, such as feeding the unhoused, engaging in social service work, and caring for the sick. Just as charity is rooted in a nondual conception of love, these acts can be seen in reciprocal terms, as people become dignified by receiving *and* by providing care to others.

Pure Love and the Little Way

As a child, Thérèse felt great sympathy for the poor and the suffering, and she expressed a strong sense of charity and generosity. In *Story of a Soul* Thérèse recalled how, when she and her family would go out walking on Sundays, "We frequently met poor people on these long walks, and it was always little Thérèse who was put in charge of bringing them alms, which made her quite happy." Thérèse's mother Zélie was known to feed beggars, and Thérèse herself recounted how, "During the walks I took with Papa, he loved to have me bring alms to the poor we met on the way." In one of their outings, Thérèse encountered a man on crutches who did not consider himself sufficiently impoverished to accept the coin that she offered. Thérèse's heart was so moved by this encounter that she became determined to offer him something of value. Thérèse resolved to pray for him on her First Communion Day, when "we can obtain whatever we ask for." While she was only six at the time, Thérèse recalled: "I kept my promise five years later, and I hope God answered the prayer He inspired me to direct to Him in favor of one of His suffering members."[2]

Later in life, Thérèse adopted a personal coat of arms that bore resonant words from Saint John of the Cross's *Spiritual Canticle*: "Love is repaid by Love alone." Thérèse also quoted from this source in *Story of a Soul* when she observed that "the smallest act of PURE LOVE is of more value to [the Church] than all other works together."[3] While Thérèse adopted the motto with a flourish of pageantry, in her writings she repeatedly emphasized her own humbleness and smallness. The "little way" centers on such themes of modesty, humility, attention to the ordinary details of life, and expressions of kindness that are offered without expectation of anything in return. When commenting on these subjects in *Story of a Soul*, Thérèse referenced the Book of Matthew (6: 3): "God made me feel that true glory is that which will last eternally, and to reach it, it isn't necessary to perform striking works but to hide oneself and practice virtue in such a way that the left hand knows not what the right is doing."[4]

Thérèse put this ethic into practice at the convent at Lisieux. Her vision of the "little way" included performing small services for the ill and the elderly, including caring for disagreeable people and suffering souls. At the convent, Thérèse attended to the needs of a difficult elderly nun, including walking her from one room to another and cutting her food for her. While performing such humble acts, Thérèse received a luminous vision of charity. As she wrote, "I cannot express in words what happened in my soul; what I know is that the Lord illumined it with rays of *truth* which so surpassed the dark brilliance of earthly feasts that I could not believe my happiness. Ah! I would not have exchanged the ten minutes employed in carrying out my humble office of charity to enjoy a thousand years of worldly feasts."[5]

Broad Shoulders and a Servant's Heart: Visions of Love and Caring

Related themes of compassion, charity, and service arise throughout end-of-life narratives. One day I met a middle-aged woman who was in full contact isolation as she suffered from an extremely rare and aggressive form of leukemia. The woman had lost much of her motor function, and her face and body were covered in a bright red rash. Despite the severity of her condition and her correspondingly dire prognosis, the woman was lucid and thoughtful as she shared her images of service and grace. Referencing the biblical verse of Philippians (4: 7), she described

A Vision of Love and Caring

I go to a small church,
And we work with a lot of senior citizens.
So many of our seniors have been left alone,
Because their families are gone,
Or, because they don't have families.
So, we reach out to them.

I can't do that any more
Because I have a terminal condition.
But, I'm at peace with it.

I see visions of love and caring.
I said to my daughter, "I don't understand it."
And she said, "It's because that's the life you have lived."
It is the peace that passes all understanding.
It's the peace
And the love.

Another woman sat up in bed, surrounded by friends. As she spoke, I learned of the extensive volunteer work she had performed earlier in life, acts that created dignity and independence among vulnerable populations. This woman was extremely slight and frail, and her voice was so soft I had to lean in closely to hear her words. I smiled when I wrote the paradoxical title of her story, which referenced not her physical form but the stature of her character:

Broad Shoulders

I like helping people.
I like people to be comfortable.
I try to care for people as much as I can.
I have broad shoulders.

In Nigeria, I trained people to train people.
I like people to be independent,
And to have something that they can call their own.
Above all, I like all those around me to be free.

Sometimes families will honor a person at the end of life by describing the acts of care and kindness they performed on behalf of others. The adult daughter of an elderly man characterized her father as having

A Servant's Heart

My dad loves unconditionally.
He has a servant's heart.

He liked to take care of others.
He saw the positive in people that,
Maybe, others didn't see.
And he always had faith in someone's ability
To make better choices.

He's a caregiver,
And he loved people.

Drawing on language that resonates with Thérèse's "little way," another man honored his elderly mother by describing her life as a vision of

Simplicity

My mother is always grateful and always positive.
She always let people in the house.
She's always very welcoming,
Very warm and kind.

She's the type of person who would cook for people.
My mother was a caretaker for the elderly,
And she is very close to God.

We're Roman Catholics.
She was always willing to help and to give,
Even when her own means were limited.

She's a very simple person.
So many people have come to her during this difficult time,
Because she is wonderful.

While working in Acute Palliative Care, I have repeatedly witnessed the ways in which seemingly small things can mean almost everything. We can never fully know the depths of what someone or something can mean to another. And, no matter how much we do know, the reality can always be deeper—and more beautiful—than we ever could have imagined.

She Came Into My Life: There Are No Such Things as Small Things

Just as facing the end of life can be a humbling and debilitating experience, moments of care and normalcy can be extremely powerful. Such ordinary moments can generate extraordinary insights because they demonstrate the great value of the "small things" that show us our humanity. One man expressed his heartfelt appreciation for the unexpected assistance he received from a friend:

She Came Into My Life

She came into my life
And started picking up the pieces,
Just helping out,
Without ever being asked to.
She didn't have to do that.
She did it because it needed to be done.
I was shocked that she would do this,
But it was powerful for her to lend a hand.
Little things are so significant.

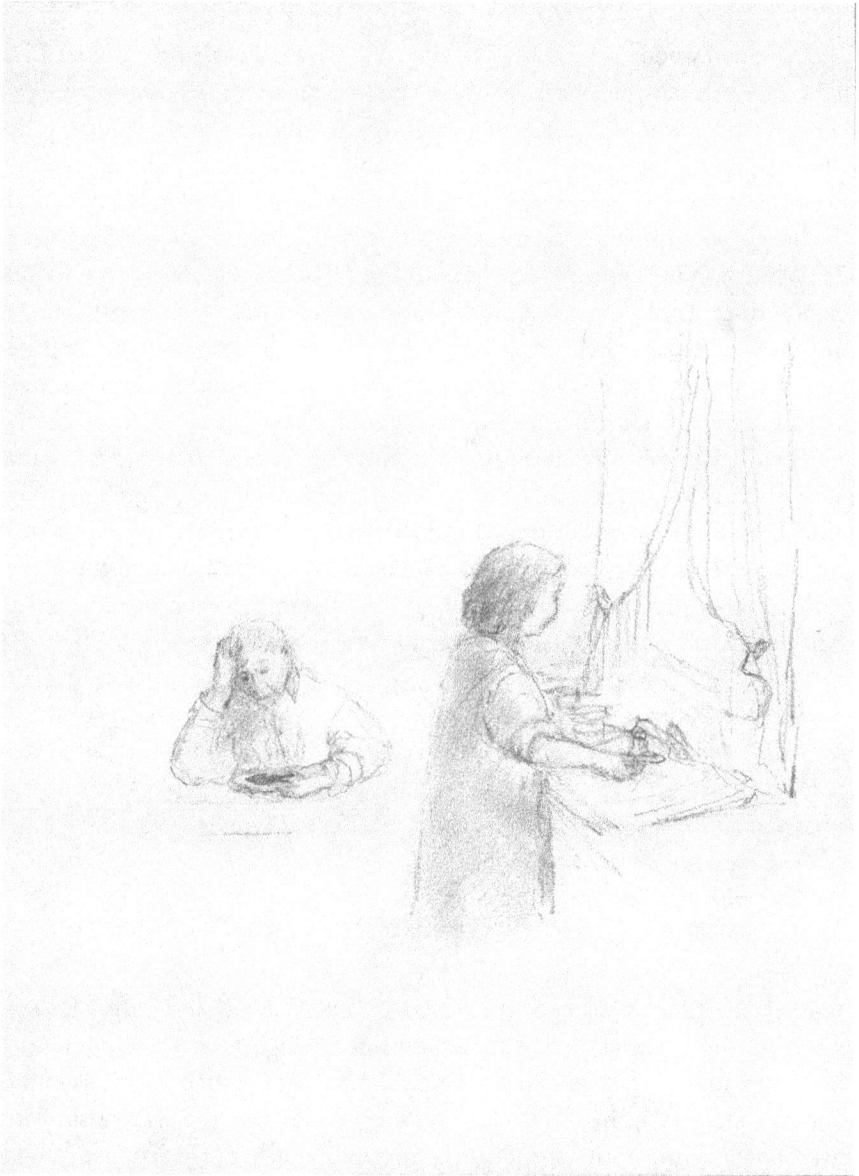

Figure 13: Lyn Smallwood, *She Came Into My Life*, 2021, graphite on white Strathmore drawing paper

Lyn Smallwood's soft pencil drawing, *She Came Into My Life* (Figure 13), depicts such small yet monumental gestures of care. In this intimate image, an older man sits at a kitchen table, holding his head in a weary gesture as he contemplates a plate of food. A woman in the foreground appears as a cheerful, sturdy presence who does the dishes while facing a bright kitchen window. The image looks like an ordinary genre scene, like a familiar image of everyday life. While nothing appears to be special about it, when the image is viewed in relation to the man's narrative, we begin to see what might otherwise remain unseen. We discern the larger patterns embedded within the moment, and we recognize the magnitude of seemingly small acts of care and kindness, where nothing is too humble to be an embodiment of grace.

Both end-of-life narratives and Thérèse's writings emphasize the importance of performing such small acts with great love. One day I met a lovely middle-aged woman who suffered from an aggressive brain tumor. This was a relatively recent diagnosis, and the woman cried as she recounted the many hardships that this illness caused her and her young children. Amidst these difficulties, the woman spoke proudly of her teenage daughter:

> *She's the biggest help I have.*
> *I don't know what I would do without her.*
> *She does everything.*
> *She does all the little things I need,*
> *And she keeps such a good attitude.*
> *I'm proud and I'm blessed,*
> *And I know it.*

Another day I met a woman who had experienced a very hard life. She was now adjusting to the news that she suffered from Stage 3 renal carcinoma and that her treatment options were extremely limited. At the time she didn't know how much longer she had left to live, yet she was clearly not ready to assimilate this difficult diagnosis or to accept the possibility of her own passing. While negotiating these complicated issues, she found that her perspective was rapidly shifting. As she said:

> *When you get sick, everything's different.*
> *Now I'm looking at life a little differently,*
> *And respecting it,*
> *Because I'm in this situation.*
> *Little things now mean everything,*
> *And everything matters.*

Another young woman with advanced lymphoma lay paralyzed in bed, unable to move from the waist down. Yet she was smiling because, a little later that afternoon, she was expecting a visit from her sons. Her younger boy was in pre-school, while her "big boy" was in elementary school. While she was realistic enough to know that this scenario was unlikely, this young mother still longed to go outdoors and kick the soccer ball around the park with her children. As she said:

> *I don't know what God has in store for me.*
> *But I do know that there will never be another "normal day" again.*
> *Should God grant me the use of my feet and the ability to wiggle my toes,*
> *I'll never see that as a small thing again.*

When we recognize the little things that are so significant, we find ourselves recalling incidental yet important moments filled with love, support, and comfort. The end of life can be an exceptional teacher of this transformational perspective.

Performing Little Services Without Any Recognition

As she was preparing to enter the Carmel, Thérèse performed "little services without any recognition" for those around her. When she arrived at the convent, Thérèse recalled how "I applied myself to practicing little virtues, not having the capability of practicing the great," and so instead she provided "little services" to her fellow nuns.[6] These acts included making a conscious effort to see the good in people, especially when it was difficult to do so. Through spiritual reflection, Thérèse came to understand that "charity consists in bearing with the faults of others, in not being surprised at their weakness, in being edified by the smallest acts of virtue we see them practice." This led to her desire to take action: "I must seek out in recreation, on free days, the company of Sisters who are the least agreeable to me in order to carry out with regard to these wounded souls the office of the good Samaritan. A word, an amiable smile, often suffice to make a sad soul bloom."[7]

On another day I visited with a middle-aged woman whose husband was nearly nonresponsive due to his metastatic liver cancer. As the woman reflected on the man's life and legacy, her thoughts kept returning to how her husband worked for several decades in an institutional setting, caring for mentally challenged adults. As the woman described her husband's gentle approach, she recalled the many things he did by approaching people

As A Friend

My husband is a very caring man.
He worked with mentally challenged individuals.
He loved these individuals.
He started out as an aide, and over the years,
He was promoted to administration.
He even worked as an investigator,
Both for these people and for their families.
If they had any concerns, they went to him.

You have to have patience to deal with a mentally challenged person.
You have to have a lot of understanding,
And it's not easy.
You have to accept them as they are.

Sometimes people can be aggressive.
The patients would stop their aggression if they saw my husband.
It's as if he's talking to them—
Not as a patient—
But as a friend.
And they responded to him,
And respected him.
And of course,
I am so proud.

A similar story arose the day I worked with a family whose middle-aged daughter lay in bed, dying of breast cancer. While the woman was sedated and only minimally responsive, several of her senior family members gathered to attend her passing. Everyone emphasized the ways in which the woman spent her life serving the underserved. Their narrative reflects the family's deep spiritual belief that

God Gave Her to Us

My daughter is very giving and caring and protective.
Her heart is open, and she is receptive to good.
For many years, she worked at a home for people who are disabled.
She lived right there in the house with them.

*She was **their back**.*
She would take them shopping, and she carried them back and forth on trips.
She was a very good caregiver.
She was one of those people who could do it with a smile.
We're a close knit family.
Everybody is for everybody.
Her strength came from family.
God gave her to us.

God Put Me In His Arms: Caring for the Sick and Dying

At the convent, Thérèse served as a caregiver for the sick and dying. A few years after joining the convent, Thérèse found herself living amidst a deadly influenza epidemic. This was the "Russian pandemic" of 1889 to 1892. Named for its original outbreak in St. Petersburg, the virus spread rapidly across Eurasia and the Americas. As one of only a handful of healthy individuals in her community, Thérèse assumed substantial duties while those around her grew extremely ill and several passed away. Although still a teenager, she helped to prepare the burials of her fellow nuns. When later reflecting on this experience, Thérèse found herself at a loss for words. As she wrote: "Never could I describe all the things I witnessed, what life appeared to be like, and everything that happened." Even as "Death reigned supreme," Thérèse recalled feeling a sense of divine protection during this period of sadness and struggle. In particular, she felt herself surrounded by a divine presence that removed fear and provided strength. Thus even in the most difficult circumstances, Thérèse "felt that God was watching over us."[8]

Years later, when facing the end of her own life, Thérèse noted how easy it is for the sick to become discouraged. For this reason she instructed her fellow nuns to "pray for the poor sick who are dying. If you only knew what happens! How little it takes to lose one's patience! You must be kind towards all of them without exception. I would not have believed this formerly."[9] To her sister Marie, Thérèse further expressed her belief that people are drawn to healthcare professions "through the attraction of grace." She then expressed her wish to have served as a care provider for a nun in the infirmary who required much attention. Quoting Matthew (25: 36), Thérèse reflected, "How happy I would have been to be her infirmarian. This would have cost me much according to my natural inclinations, but it seems to me I would have taken care of her with so much love, because I think of what Our Lord said: 'I was sick and you visited me.'"[10]

Such acts of giving and receiving care emerged the day I met a middle-aged woman who was planning to bring her adult daughter home for hospice care. The woman was a practical nurse, and during our visit she spoke about her dedication to her profession and the significance of working with her hands. As she proudly told me:

They've Touched a Lot of People

I love nursing,
And I love taking care of people.
I trust in God,
And I'm learning to be stronger.

I'm a hard worker,
And I give care to my patients.
I know they miss me
Because I keep them laughing all the time.
I don't mind doing anything for them—
Bathing them, dressing them, feeding them, or wiping up.
I'm learning to be patient
And take one day at a time.

When I first got into nursing,
I felt like my hands weren't good enough.
Now, after all these years,
I can say that it's good to be of help to someone.
These hands have seen a lot of hard work,
And they've touched a lot of people.

Another day I met a middle-aged woman who sat stiffly propped up in a chair, gingerly attempting to eat some soft food. Despite her pronounced lymph-edema and her numerous facial tumors, a soft light came into her eyes as she described a spiritual image of being

In His Arms

I think I have the best doctors in the world.
If there was a way to save my life,
They would have done it.

These doctors are passionate about their patients.
I have a good team behind me.

My doctor takes the time to explain what's going on.
He asks me if I understand what he's telling me,
Before I ever leave the room.
Then, both of us are almost in tears.
That kind of care is amazing.

Sometimes I think
God put me in his arms.

I Don't Know How I've Touched You

When a person is gravely ill, their world can become extremely constrained. In these very limited circumstances, seemingly small gestures of kindness and care can be monumental. These themes arose the day I visited with a fragile elderly woman who spent her entire professional career as a nurse. Despite her advanced neurocranial cancer, the woman remained lucid throughout the visit. When I first entered the room, the woman was admittedly very anxious. It was clear that she was not only experiencing physical pain in her extremities, but that inwardly, she was mourning the loss of her mobility and her motor functions. At her request, I shifted the position of her feet and placed a blanket under her ankles. As we visited, the woman's pain began to subside. Ultimately, we produced a very moving artwork:

I Don't Know How I've Touched You

I am a nurse.
I can't do anything else.
I love people.
I have seen how nurses are caring, loving, and compassionate.
They think, "It doesn't matter what this person is doing to me.
It's not about me.
It's that they are hurting.
What can I do to relieve their pain?"

Being a nurse means that I care about you.

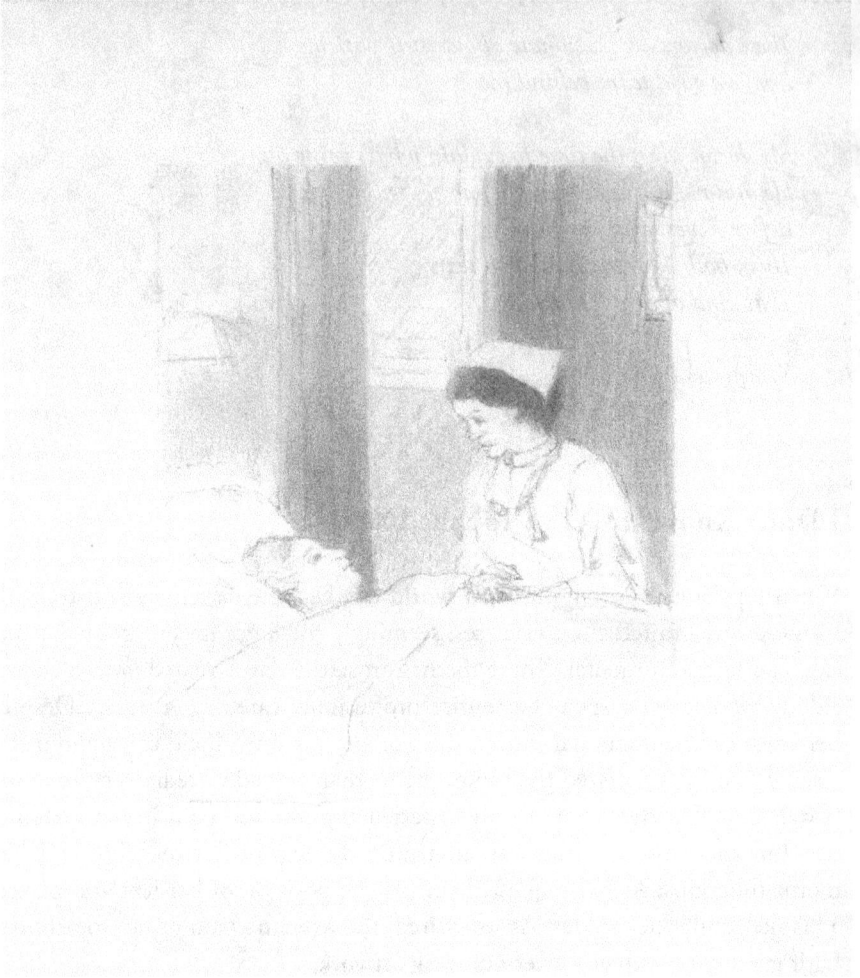

Figure 14: Lyn Smallwood, *I Don't Know How I've Touched You*, 2016, graphite on white Arches paper

I deeply care about you.
I want to ease your pain.
You can get mad at me.
But, I want to take your pain away.
This makes me feel I've succeeded in my life.

I don't know how I've touched you.
I don't even know what that means.
But, I know I've been successful.

Lyn Smallwood's illustration, *I Don't Know How I've Touched You* (Figure 14), depicts one person kindly attending to the needs of another. A nurse in a traditional white uniform and cap, with a stethoscope hanging around her neck, takes the hand of a bedridden patient. This image shows how providing skilled nursing care entails both practical knowledge and a tender personal touch. The artwork is marked by such a sense of reciprocity, as the two women talk quietly and look directly into one another's eyes.

After I read the words aloud, the woman and I held hands for a few minutes while she cried softly. She loved the artwork, and she generously told me that the narrative "helped me to see the meaning and purpose of my life." I assured her that the words were all her own, and that she did all the hard work and heavy lifting. The woman then asked me what drew me to palliative care. I described my work as an Artist In Residence and a professor at Rice University, and how I teach many students who, one day, will become healthcare professionals. I also briefly described my books on the end of life, and I expressed my hope that the stories will contribute to larger conversations concerning the ways in which humanistic perspectives can help to shape practices of care. The woman not only gave permission to share her story, but she went on to voice a message for all of the current and future healthcare professionals who will read her words:

That's What Mattered

I want the students to know that they can be successful.
They don't have to do any great thing.
But, they have to know they have to be there for the patient.
They don't always have to fix things.
They have to take care of the little things,
And to be surprised by how powerful this is.

> *I've had so many people come say*
> *It was the little things—*
> *Like holding my hand—*
> *That got me through the big things.*
> *Knowing that somebody cared—*
> *That's what mattered.*

Hearing this story, you may come to see that you can never fully know how you've touched another person, even as you know that you were present, and that you cared—and that's what mattered.

Medical Pedagogy and Patient-Centered Care

The nurse's artwork speaks eloquently to the importance of maintaining a humanistic perspective when confronting pronounced suffering. While such stories are for everybody, I have found that the narratives are especially valuable when teaching pre-medical and medical students, and when addressing Continuing Medical Education (CME) audiences. At the undergraduate level, students repeatedly stress that, in the standard curricula, so much material is delivered as information that there is often little opportunity to reflect on issues philosophically, or to see how they relate to one's own life experience. Throughout my teaching I emphasize the need to integrate rigorous analytical approaches with lived human experiences and with a deeply humanistic conceptual framework.

After the students graduate, they often contact me because they have witnessed something that disturbs them greatly. Within their medical training, these experiences are not limited to interactions with cancer patients. Oh no—such deeply traumatic sights can arise within the anatomy lab, the operating room, the burn unit, or during a psychiatry rotation. Again and again, my former students will recount their intense interactions with people who are staring directly into the abyss of pain and suffering, terror and death. After listening closely, I remind them of the gift of their presence, especially in these extremely difficult circumstances, and I advise them to be aware of whatever arises and to acknowledge it fully. I remind them that there are no such things as small things, and that little things may hold a world of meaning and value in ways that they can just never know. One can never underestimate the importance of accompaniment, of listening to and witnessing the presence of another. Sometimes the key is to look for the transformational element in the person's story. Whatever the circumstance, I emphasize the bravery that they exhibit by remaining present, and I ask them to consider why all of this touches them so deeply.

Related issues arise among CME audiences. When I speak to these groups, they routinely express a desire for greater integration of the arts and the humanities with science and medicine, and they welcome opportunities for further conversations. They also report that learning about these subjects will impact their healthcare practices by increasing their sense of humility, curiosity, perception, gratitude, and humanitarianism. Similarly, one of the Fellows who shadowed me on the Acute Palliative Care Unit observed that my activities engage a reciprocal dynamic between giving and taking. As I work with people, they give me their stories, and I give them back their own words as poetic narratives. In contrast, so much of the physician's work is about taking—taking inventory of a person's pain, their symptoms, and their worries, so that the healthcare provider may relieve the burdens of suffering.[11] When viewed from this perspective, much of the work of the clinical team is subtractive, while the work of the literary artist is additive. At the same time, these seemingly opposite processes of giving and taking defy easy categorization. As I visit with people and listen closely to their stories, I may help to take away the sense that they are not being heard, or that they have nothing of value to offer. Just as these creative interactions can engender an enhanced sense of presence, so too does the work of the healthcare provider. By easing or removing symptoms that cause distress, pain, or suffering, the healthcare provider performs a valuable affirmation of the person's presence.

Related insights were expressed by a fourth-year medical student who shadowed me for several weeks on the Acute Palliative Care Inpatient Unit. At the end of this experience, she emphasized the ways in which patients' voices can fill crucial gaps in medical school pedagogy. In particular, she noted that healthcare professionals who routinely deal with death rarely discuss it. Yet engaging in artistic work, and hearing the actual voices of people facing the end of life, can prepare medical students to think about death, which represents a vital step in preparing them to actually discuss the subject with vulnerable patients who may struggle with accepting a poor prognosis. She also noted that producing poetic narratives can demonstrate a sense of empathy and compassion that provides family support, a quality that can be especially valuable to meeting the needs of both patients and caregivers. She observed that such responsiveness can be extremely empowering and play a valuable role in patient-centered care.[12]

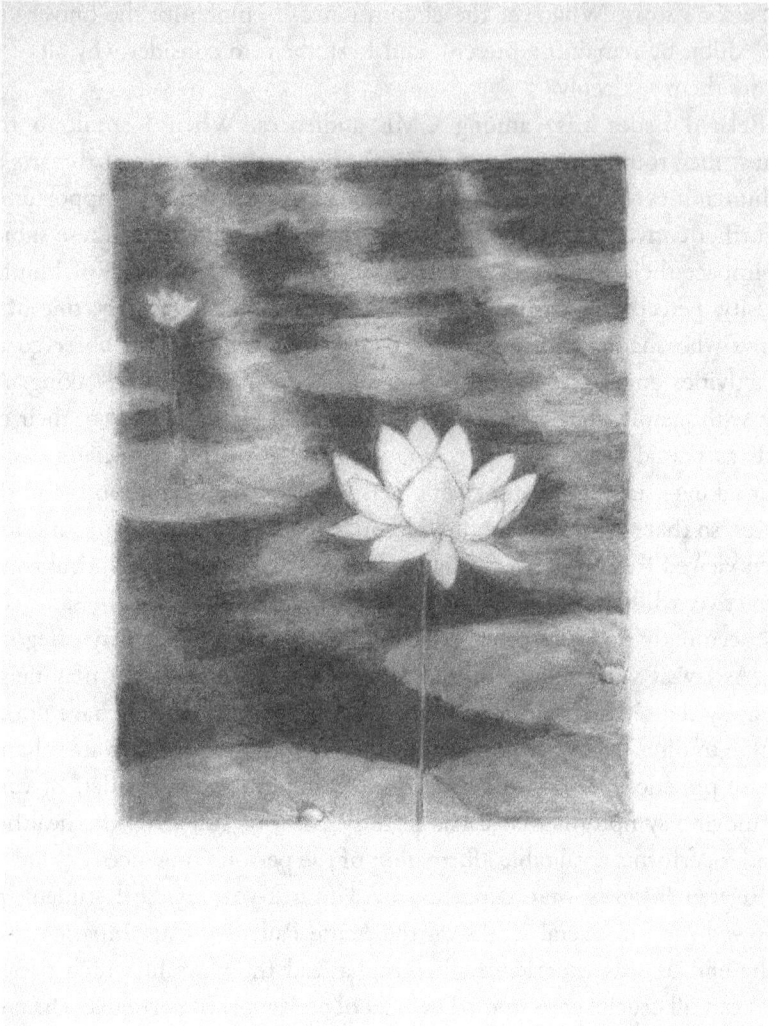

Figure 15: Lyn Smallwood, *Lotus: As Pure as the First*, 2015, graphite on white Arches paper

Lotus, as Pure as the First: Insights for Healthcare Professionals

One day I met a delicate woman who identified as Buddhist, and who shared a powerful story that engaged conceptions of purity and loss, hope and faith, death and ongoing life. This woman had only been diagnosed a few months earlier. The frailty of her emaciated frame was pronounced, and a drainage tube extended from her nose to the suction device positioned at the head of her bed. The woman was originally from China, and she had young children at home. This woman had important things to say about medicine, especially how, after her initial diagnosis, she wanted to be tough and not take pain medicine, and how this decision robbed her of precious days with her family. When I asked the woman about what she felt was important for people to know, she responded:

> Doctors need to know what is humanly tolerable, not just in the body. Most doctors treat the disease. The disease is a physical organism. In this hospital, they treat humans with the disease. It's the human that is important. It's feelings, with spiritual needs. People encourage you to keep fighting, to fight the cancer. To know when to surrender is also a fight. Also the hospital is an international center, and it is helpful for doctors to have background on where patients come from, and what is important to them.

When I initially approached the woman's room, I wasn't sure if she would want—or be able—to work together, as she seemed so weak and drowsy. Yet as our visit unfolded, the woman came into greater strength and energy. At the end of our time together she called the visit an unexpected gift, and she emphasized the beauty of the heart, which she saw reflected in her artwork:

Lotus: As Pure as the First

My image is of flowers,
Of lotus.
It grows out of the mud.
But it's so white,
So pure.
The lotus is always important for me.
It's just the pureness.

I want the world to be like that,

With not many evil things.
Just the pureness.
I like the water that collects on the lotus leaves.
It's shining.
I want my young children
To grow up to be as pure as possible,
Not contaminated by the world,
But to keep as clean as possible.
This is something very difficult,
To stay as yourself in the world.
To stay as a child in this world.

Children have to grow.
They don't have control over this.
They have to grow.
Eventually, they grow up, and they die,
And there will be new life again.
Hopefully, as pure as the first.

Lyn Smallwood's soft pencil illustration (Figure 15) is as complex and delicate as the woman's story. In this image, water lilies float gently on a pond, where they are framed by the mutually reflective surfaces of the water and the sky. In the immediate foreground, an open white lotus appears in full bloom. Much as in the woman's story, a brightly shining drop of water has collected at the center of the flower's leaves. The white lotus appears as an embodiment of purity and the renewal of life amidst the transient conditions of a floating world. This tender image is also paradoxical. It provides something concrete for the viewer's eye and mind to hold onto as the world slips away and familiar images of life transform before us. By encompassing these themes, the flower is a small thing that can mean almost everything.

Notes

1. Thomas R. Nevin notes that Thérèse may not have been the originator of the "little way" for which she is so well known. Instead, this concept may have been inspired by a young Parisian woman named Berthe Vosgelin whose devotional writings Thérèse's sister, Marie, may have given her to copy as a child. The relevant passage in Vosgelin's writings concerns walking with "a steady step on my little way" of life. Nevin further notes that such themes are consistent with the Carmelite approach of achieving sanctity through "the faithful accomplishment of little things." See Nevin, *Thérèse of Lisieux*, 44–45, 115.
2. Quoted in *Story of a Soul*, 278, 72.
3. Quoted in *Story of a Soul*, 197.
4. Quoted in *Story of a Soul*, 30, 38.
5. Quoted in *Story of a Soul*, 197.
6. Quoted in *Story of a Soul*, 143, 159.
7. Quoted in *Story of a Soul*, 220–23, 246–47.
8. Quoted in *Story of a Soul*, 63, 171–72.
9. Quoted in *St. Thérèse of Lisieux*, 130, 132.
10. Quoted in *St. Thérèse of Lisieux*, 156, 242.
11. I am grateful to Dr. Astrid Grouls for sharing these observations, in correspondence with the author, September 1, 2019.
12. I am grateful to Dr. Amberly Orr, who expressed her observations on the shadowing experience in her final essay, "Lessons on Dying: What Patients Taught Me That Was Missing From Medical School."

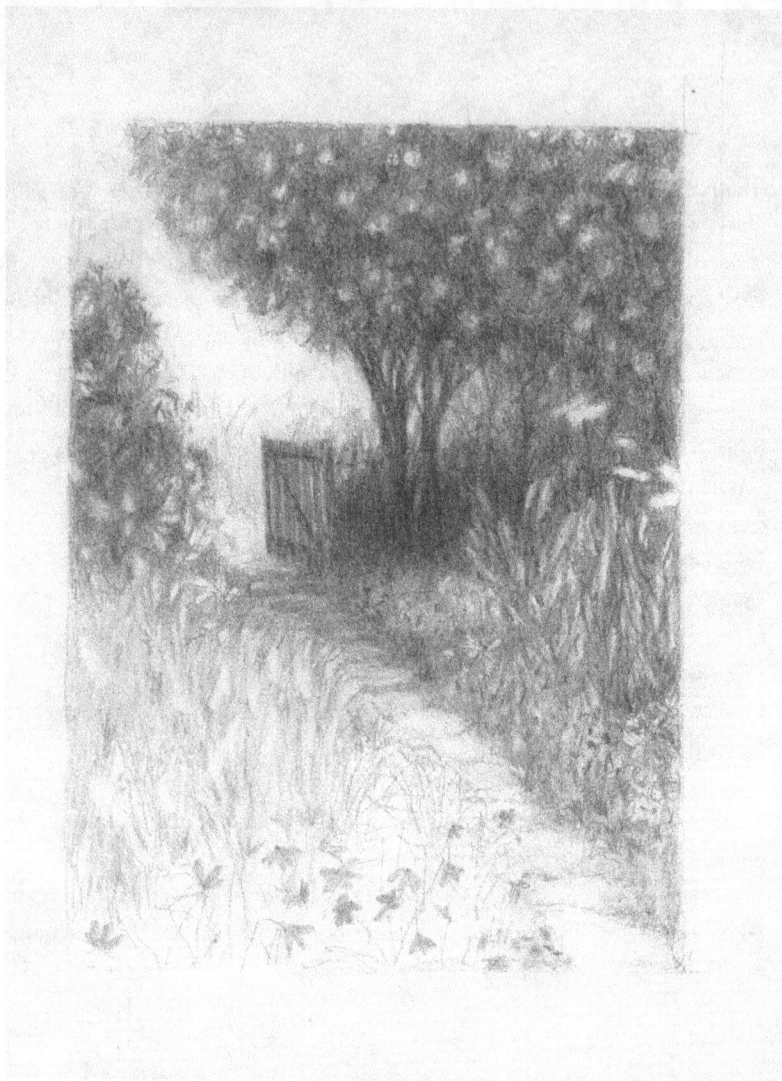

Figure 16: Lyn Smallwood, *The Garden Is Full of Little Things*, 2012, graphite on white Arches paper

Chapter Four

The Garden in the Garden: The Spiritual Significance of Flowers

Once Again, Why Small Things Matter

One of the most powerful lessons I ever learned in palliative care came from an elderly lady who appeared to have almost nothing. With great delicacy *and* great power, this woman showed me that transforming a person's perspective can transform their sense of reality, and in turn, that a transformed vision of reality can transform a person's perspective.

The woman had been brought to the hospital in the middle of the night, from out of state, and in a great deal of pain. Now at the very end of her life, her advanced liver cancer was evident in her pronounced jaundice, her generally weakened condition, and the frail bone structure that protruded beneath her emaciated frame. Because of her emergency hospital admission, the woman had not had time to pack even the most basic necessities, such as a toothbrush, toothpaste, or hand lotion. When we first met, the woman asked me quietly if I had any of these items with me. At the moment, I hadn't, so I went down to the hospital gift shop and purchased a toothbrush and some trial-size tubes of toiletries. A little while later, when I presented the woman with these modest items, she accepted them with such surprise that I was nearly knocked off my feet. As the frail woman reached out to receive the toothbrush, our hands briefly touched, and I felt such a surge of gratitude flowing from her that words failed me entirely. For a moment, all I could do was stand there with tears in my eyes as I smiled quietly and acknowledged her thanks.

In the intensity of that instant, the woman taught me a powerful lesson that I will never forget, namely: *Things that are so small that they seem to mean almost nothing can mean almost everything, and conversely, things that are so large, valuable, and important that they seem to mean everything can mean almost nothing at all.* Just as I gifted the woman with a handful of incidental items, she taught me a valuable lesson concerning the paradox of presence. She showed me that great delicacy and great power are neither mutually exclusive nor categorically oppositional, but rather, that these qualities can deepen, heighten, and strengthen one another. All of which is to say that, in our brief exchange, everything was turned on its head, and yet everything was in its proper place. Just as the frail woman's grace and strength nearly overwhelmed me, she brought me to a place beyond language—a place of understanding that lay beyond words.

This initial encounter set the tone for the artwork we produced a little later that afternoon. As the woman and I visited for about an hour and a half, she spoke at length about her home in Louisiana and her garden in the country. She became so immersed in these topics that, despite her extreme weakness, she insisted on making a small but detailed pencil sketch of the garden's site plan. After describing the minute details of the various plants that filled her garden, the woman reflected on the larger meanings she found in this peaceful place:

The Garden Is Full of Little Things

I have a garden,
And I enjoy being outside with the flowers.
I love pulling the weeds from the wild flowers,
And doing anything
To make the yard pretty.

I have pink and red roses and raspberry crepe myrtles,
And ground covers with impatiens,
And we have little jalapeno peppers.
I don't know all the names of the flowers,
But I go to the flower shop and look around.

I've always wanted a garden,
And my husband carved it out for me.
He put in some flagstones
All the way to the gate.

When I'm in the garden,
I don't think of anything
But being out there,

And working in my flowers.

You pull the weeds, and you plant.
What grows, grows.
What survives, survives.

The garden is full of little things.
It's an awful lot of work,
And there are lots of things I had to just let go of.
But it's what I've always dreamed of doing:
Caring for little things,
Like God says in the Bible.

Lyn Smallwood's illustration, *The Garden Is Full of Little Things* (Figure 16), displays a curving flagstone path bordered with flowering rose bushes and crepe myrtle trees set amidst lush summer grasses. Much like the woman's story, the pencil drawing evokes a scene of luxurious abundance. The densely clustered foliage of the tree canopy both contrasts with, and counterbalances, the lightness of the foreground, where borders of wildflowers and strands of tall grasses flank a gently winding path that leads to an open garden gate, a sight that evokes the ambivalent possibilities of coming and going. The hinged gate swings forward to extend invitingly to a space beyond the garden, an opening that is not yet fully visible, a clearing that is filled with light.

When describing the significance of the garden, the woman paraphrased the biblical verse of Luke 16:10: "Whoever can be trusted with very little can also be trusted with much, and whoever is dishonest with very little will also be dishonest with much."[1] Like so many of the artworks that appear in this chapter, in this story the garden serves as a portal to the sacred, while the sacred serves as a portal to the garden.[2] Just as the woman observed that gardening involves "pulling the weeds from the wild flowers," she emphasized the need to distinguish her priorities so that she could identify the things that she "had to let go of," and the things she could continue to nurture and cherish. This conscious sense of stewardship enabled her to practice a very beautiful and difficult paradox, that of holding on by letting go.

The Uniqueness of Souls: Thérèse on the Book of Nature

Just as people at the end of life will often invest the natural landscape with such transcendent associations, these themes represent a leitmotif in the writings of Thérèse of Lisieux. Thérèse is popularly known as the Little Flower, and images of flowers appear throughout the writings of this saint. Among other meanings, flowers serve as devotional offerings that connect the material and the spiritual worlds while linking conceptions of simplicity and profundity through the realms of life and death.[3] Resonating with the opening story, Thérèse also described how she was taught "the way of becoming *holy* through fidelity in little things."[4]

For Thérèse, colorful fields of wildflowers inspired thoughts of divine presence, and she characterized such scenes as heaven scattering masterpieces on earth. In one of her best known formulations, Thérèse commented on the ways in which flowers can be seen as metaphors for human souls. Emphasizing the magnitude of seemingly small things, Thérèse began her spiritual autobiography by raising the fundamental question of why some individuals seem to be favored in life, while others face great hardships and struggles. She presented her insights as a kind of dialogue with divine presence:

> He set before me the book of nature; I understood how all the flowers He has created are beautiful, how the splendor of the rose and the whiteness of the lily do not take away the perfume of the little violet or the delightful simplicity of the daisy. I understood that if all flowers wanted to be roses, nature would lose her springtime beauty, and the fields would no longer be decked out with little wild flowers. And so it is in the world of souls.[5]

Thérèse then observed that "since the nature of love is to humble oneself," it is to the most vulnerable beings "that God deigns to lower Himself. These are the wild flowers whose simplicity attracts Him. When coming down in this way, God manifests His infinite grandeur."[6] Just as Thérèse compared human souls to flowers, she saw the heaven world descending to earth as a gift of love.

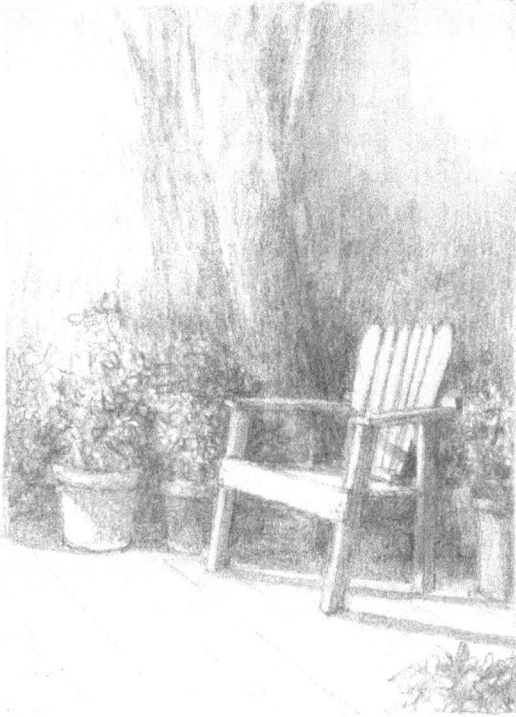

Figure 17: Lyn Smallwood, *Jade*, 2012, graphite on white Arches paper

Jade: Talking with God in the Garden

In Thérèse's writings, flowers repeatedly serve as intermediate presences between the earth and the heavens. In so doing, they appear to embody the intrinsic value—and even, the singular grandeur—of ordinary life. I have often seen these themes arise in palliative care. A few months after I met the elderly woman who described the ways in which her garden is "full of little things," I encountered another very sweet, very frail woman who also loved to garden. Lying quietly in bed with large hollow eyes and deeply sunken cheekbones, the woman looked as though she had already passed out of this life. She was extremely weak and her voice was nearly inaudible, yet she brightened visibly when she heard that an artist was there, and she wanted to talk about her love of the garden. While the flower garden in the opening story is a large, bright, open space in the countryside, the palette of the second garden is decidedly more austere. The subdued design of the woman's urban patio garden was distinguished by the thick, round, dark green leaves of her prized jade plants, the earthen warmth of their terracotta pots, and the reddish-brown bricks that formed the base of the courtyard. In language that was correspondingly spare and restrained, the woman described her small garden as an enclosed sanctuary filled with personal and spiritual meanings:

Jade

I love my garden.
There's a dark green plant with thick leaves
That grows all over the garden.
They are jade plants.
I never had them grow until the last several years,
And then they took off and started to grow.

I have a brick patio, and I loved sitting out there,
Especially in the evenings, when it wasn't too hot.
It was peaceful,
And it was a good time to commune with God.

After I read the story aloud, the woman nodded and affirmed, "Those are my thoughts." She then told me that she had painted a little, earlier in her life, when she was a young married woman. When I asked her about the types of subjects that she painted, not surprisingly, she replied, "Things in my garden."

Lyn Smallwood's pencil illustration, *Jade* (Figure 17), displays a complementary sense of simplicity and directness. The drawing depicts a small, rectangular patio garden whose perimeter edges are bordered by the trunks of tall trees and flourishing rows of potted jade plants. The bottom edge of the drawing is suggestively left open, as if creating space for viewers to enter. Much as in the woman's narrative, in this artwork the garden appears as a natural sanctuary. Paradoxically, this humble yet elegant scene is bright yet shaded, minimal yet flourishing. The drawing's clean lines and textured surfaces contrast the densely clustered leaves of the potted jade plants with the smooth clay bricks of the patio and the upright wooden slats of the chair on which the woman sat as she contemplated the natural world and communed with God.[7]

The Trees Appeared to Be Golden: The Metaphysics of the Natural World

As a child, Thérèse created small contemplative gardens both in the attic of her home, *Les Buissonnets*, and outdoors among the trees and flowers where she set up "little altars in a niche in the middle of the wall."[8] Thérèse also recalled how, in her youth, her father took her on fishing trips and she would "go *alone* and sit down on the grass bedecked with flowers, and then my thoughts became very profound indeed! Without knowing what it was to meditate, my soul was absorbed in real prayer."[9] In her writings Thérèse characterized gardens as uniting the domains of below and above, the intimate and the expansive, the humble and the sacred. Thérèse also described herself as a kind of artistic medium, a "paintbrush" whose life was used to illustrate the smallest details of numinous presence. She affirmed the value of such metaphorical imagery when she noted that, as human beings, "we need pictures to understand spiritual things."[10]

Later in life, as she faced serious illness, Thérèse found deep inspiration in the natural world. Thérèse told her sister Marie that

> When bending over a little, I saw through the window the setting sun that was casting its rays over nature, and the tops of the trees appeared to be golden. I said to myself: What a difference if one remains in the shadows or, on the contrary, if one exposes oneself to the sun of Love. Then we appear all golden. In reality, I am not this, and I would cease to be this immediately if I were to withdraw myself from Love.[11]

Thérèse's observations read like a spiritual parable. With characteristic humility, she describes the golden light that is available to all, like the trees that are rooted firmly in the earth yet whose tops are illuminated by radiant sunlight. People at the end of life will similarly speak with great simplicity and power when they look out their windows and describe their perceptions of the natural world as a space of radiance.

I once met a Latin American woman who was a research scientist. When I first entered the room the woman was alert, oriented, and making plans to leave with home hospice. She knew that she was dying, and she expressed great sadness that she had reached the end of her life while still only at middle age. When I first introduced myself as an Artist In Residence, the woman was very wary, and she almost declined to work with me, saying that she was in a great deal of pain. I told her that sometimes people found it helpful to work together, and that their pain eased while we talked. Would she like to give it a try? While clearly skeptical, the woman retained her demeanor as a scientist, and she said that she was open to experimentation and observation. I pulled a footstool up to her bed and I offered to hold her hand while I took down her words.

As soon as we began speaking, the woman identified her significant image. In the innocence of childhood, she had a vision of nature as a vital source of life. As she described the image, she acknowledged that she could feel her pain receding. At the end of the visit, the woman told me that she did feel better—and she kissed me and thanked me. Hearing her beautiful words read aloud, she generously gave permission to share the story. As she said, "We have to go someplace in our spirituality"—and this was her place:

I Opened the Window

I was raised in Latin America,
And my image is from my childhood.
I have just this one image, and this is it:

I was a little girl, and we had just moved to a new house.
I had a new room, and I opened the window.
It had just rained, and I could smell the rain.
It was the view of the jungle, and the smell of the rain.
The dirt was wet, and a breeze was coming in.
It was the smell of the wetness of the black dirt
And the greenery of the earth, soaked in rain.

It is something that goes together.
It goes as a whole.
You cannot describe it.
It was wonderful.
It's a part of me, still.
You smell this and you say,
"It's alive!"
And it is.

I've never felt it like that again.
I've looked for it—and, I've gotten glimpses of it—
But the purity of my eyes as a child was so intense.

With this image, you just feel alive.
You just feel like, this is where the fountain is.
This is life itself.

By drawing on this powerful childhood image, the woman told a creation story as she faced the end of her life. Another day I met a woman who described a trip that she and her husband had taken to Europe several years earlier to celebrate a significant anniversary. Among the many beautiful sights they encountered were the breathtaking colors of the Dutch flower gardens and flower markets. The woman also mentioned how much she enjoyed the photographs of flowers that decorated the walls at M.D. Anderson, and how these images brought her comfort while she spent extended time in the waiting areas. In these transitional spaces, floral imagery helped to provide a sense of grounding *and* of uplift. Conjoining these associations, the woman reflected on

The Beauty of the Tulips

For our wedding anniversary,
My husband and I travelled to Europe,
And we visited the flower gardens and the flower markets in Holland.
I love the flower photos that they have
In the waiting areas at M.D. Anderson.
In one waiting room, there is a large blown up picture
Of tulips on the wall.

While I waited for the doctor,

I got to reflect on the beautiful trip we took.
And, I got to soak in the beauty of the flowers.
I would lose myself in the vibrant colors,
And drink in the beauty of the flowers.

The flowers are a work of inspiration.
The tulips are a work of God.

For this woman, flowers and gardens appeared as symbols of comfort and uplift that evoked a paradoxical yet complementary sense of groundedness and ascension.

Everything We Love Is There: Garden Imagery and Near-Death Experiences

While working in Acute Palliative Care, I have been privileged to hear many transitional stories of worlds between worlds. One woman directed the hospital staff to rearrange the furniture so that her bed faced the large plate glass window that covered an entire wall of her room. As we spoke, the afternoon sunlight came into her eyes as the woman took in the panoramic view. She gazed directly into my eyes as she shared her vision of the heaven world, a place where

Everything We Love Is There

My husband takes good care of me.
We've been through a lot,
But we both know that everything will be fine.
We know that in our hearts.

How do I know that everything will be fine?
I died twenty years ago.
I had an asthma attack, and they brought me back.
I went to a garden, and everything was there:
Butterflies, birds, trees, flowers, and a waterfall.
I especially remember the waterfall.
It was so special.
You could feel it.

It was beautiful.

I'm going back to my garden.
Everything we love is there.

A little more than a week after our visit, the woman passed away peacefully, in that same bed, facing the picture window.

The Bright Resurrection

Another day I met a middle-aged woman who was extremely sweet, and extremely ill. Over the hiss of the high flow oxygen machine, she told me that she had "a bad scare" a few days before, and she had nearly passed away. She now only had one lung left functioning, as her metastatic cancer had spread to her lungs and bones. Yet when I walked into the room, the woman was smiling brightly. As we visited, I learned that she had spent much of her life working as a teacher and a translator, and that both she and her husband had served as Christian missionaries. Just as these elements informed her personal narrative, they directly shaped the character of her artwork. A few days before, the woman had experienced an end-of-life event in which one world merged with another. As she described the scene that she witnessed, the woman shared her vision of

The Bright Resurrection

I had a bad episode on Monday,
And my family was really scared.
My thinking at the time was:
Where are we going with this?
What will get us through this?
And the words came to me:
"The Bright Resurrection."
I was thinking of bright, colorful lights.
I like colors and brightness.
This was a flower garden type of image.

I grew up on a farm in the Midwest,
And that's the kind of picture I saw.

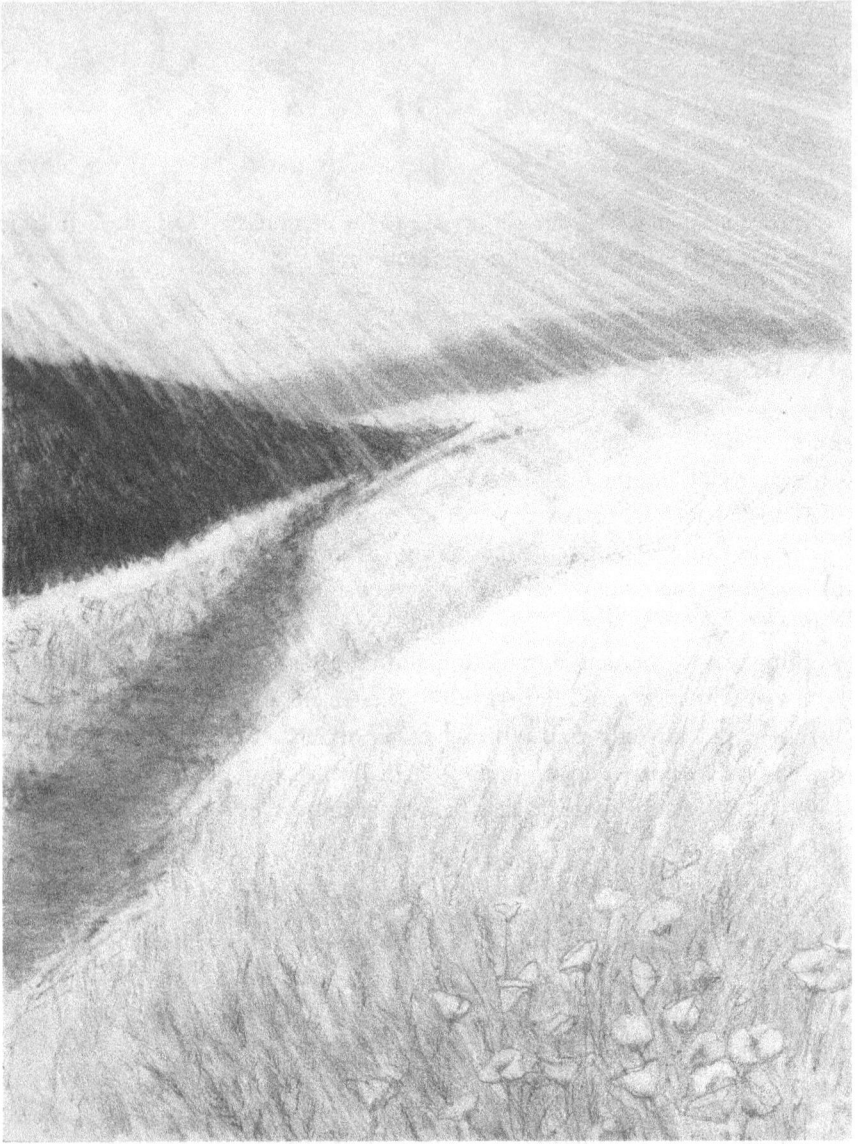

Figure 18: Lyn Smallwood, *The Bright Resurrection*, 2013, graphite on white Arches paper

The main product was, it was a dairy farm,
And the hills were fairly rolling.
That's the only place I've ever seen
The rolling waves of grain.

I'm a color person,
And I enjoyed being there.
I see bright gold in the heads of grain,
And I see the bounty.

This woman's end-of-life vision began as an otherworldly image of brightly colored lights, then it transformed into a flower garden, and ultimately, it became a lush Midwestern farm scene. Lyn Smallwood's drawing, *The Bright Resurrection* (Figure 18), presents a complementary scene of abundance. Within this layered pastoral landscape, a dark sloping hill anchors the left-hand side of the composition, while a lighter ridge appears further in the background. These contoured elements contrast with the broad expanse of the open visual field. A winding pathway cuts through a wheat field, extending diagonally through the scene while creating a narrow opening that leads the viewer's gaze into the depths of the drawing. In the foreground, ripened stalks of wheat with golden heads of grain are surrounded by the delicate blossoms of wildflowers. As the scene recedes into the background, the gently rolling wheat fields become progressively more abstract. The top third of the drawing is filled with an open sky and shafts of sunlight. The falling rays, combined with the winding path, resonate with the woman's questions of: "Where are we going with this? What will get us through this?" In short, during her near-death experience, the woman envisioned a scene of abundant life.

Related themes arose as I visited with an elderly woman who had only been admitted to the Palliative Care Inpatient Unit a few hours earlier. When I first entered the room, the patient was asleep, so I chatted quietly with the family. The woman's daughter told me how her mother loved to travel and collect antiques, and she showed me some of the paintings the family had brought with them to create a more homelike atmosphere in the hospital. Hearing us talk, the woman woke up and she asked who I was. I could see that she was on high flow oxygen and short of breath, so I knew that our encounter would be very brief. I went over to the bedside and introduced myself, and then I asked the woman if there was an image in her mind of something that held special meaning for her. She became thoughtful as she described a sense of going

Into That Light

At this moment, something that strikes me is a painting.
It's oil on canvas, and it was hanging in the bedroom.
It's a landscape with a road.
It's a happy road—
Whether you're coming or going—
And it makes me feel happy.

It just struck me as being very spiritual.
It's about walking off
Into that light.

After I read the words aloud, the woman's daughter pointed upward toward a corner of the room where the actual painting sat perched atop a wooden cabinet. Lying in her bed, the woman could look up and view the scene, and then she could look down again at all the people who had gathered at the end of her life. As we hear such stories, we too can hold multiple viewpoints simultaneously as we look up and then look down again, and we imagine walking off, into that light.

The Shower of Roses: Gifts to Others as Devotional Offerings

Of all the natural imagery that Thérèse is associated with, perhaps the best known is the "shower of roses" that she promised to send to her sisters—and to others on earth—after her passing.[12] Through this image, Thérèse anticipated a sense of her ongoing presence even as she lay in great pain and agony, surrounded by her sisters' anticipatory grief. *Butler's Lives of the Saints* puts the matter concisely by noting that, at the end of Thérèse's life,

> The spirit of prophecy seemed to come upon her, and it was now that she made those three utterances that have gone round the world. "I have never given the good God aught but love, and it is with love that He will repay. After my death I will let fall a shower of roses." "I will spend my Heaven in doing good upon earth."[13]

On June 9, 1897 Thérèse's sister Marie expressed her sorrow, to which Thérèse responded: "Oh! No, you will see ... it will be like a shower of roses. ... After my death, you will go to the mailbox, and you will find many consolations."[14] During the final weeks of her life, Thérèse's bed was placed at the center of the convent's infirmary, where she was able to see the garden in bloom. While lying there, Thérèse unpetalled roses over her crucifix, and she told her sisters to "Gather those petals, little sisters; they will help you to give pleasure later on. Do not lose one of them!"[15] Roses thus served as a symbol of Thérèse's life and as a spiritual gift for those who remained. In this way, roses have come to exemplify Thérèse's ordinariness, and her greatness.

What These Seeds Have Sown: The Things I Did Out of Love

Much as in Thérèse's writings, in end-of-life narratives flowers often appear as devotional offerings. Late one afternoon I met a woman who was being admitted to the Acute Palliative Care Inpatient Unit just as I was preparing to leave. The woman was extremely ill, and as the attendants wheeled her onto the Unit I noticed the multiple IV bags and the portable breathing apparatus that dangled at her sides. I also saw a beautiful glow in the woman's light brown eyes. Once she was settled into her room, I introduced myself and admired the flowers she had brought with her. The woman then spoke about the flowers, and she shared related images of the heaven world:

Even More Beautiful

My image is of God reaching down His hand for me.
I hope people don't think I'm giving up.
This is something that came to me,
And I knew the Lord would take care of me.

When I picture heaven,
I just picture a smiling face,
And I picture flowers,
All different kinds of flowers,
Especially roses and hydrangeas.
I love hydrangeas.
They're my very favorite.

The smiling face is Jesus saying,
"You finally got here.

You finally made it."

My garden at home is a beautiful place,
But heaven is going to be
Even more beautiful.

After I read the narrative aloud, the woman said that she loved the story, and she began to cry. She then told me that she had seen this imagery in her mind, and that she was now thinking about subjects such as this. She clearly cherished her home, her garden, and the people around her, and these images returned to her as she contemplated

The Things I Did Out of Love

Many years ago,
I had a friend whose house burned down,
And she lost all her clothing.
I made a dress for this woman on my sewing machine.
This was a long time ago, and I had forgotten all about it.
But recently, this lady wrote me a letter
Reminding me about this and thanking me.
This brought me to tears.
I'm thinking a lot about things like this now,
The things I did, not to be thanked.
Now I think about all of the good things,
The things I did out of love.

Those are the seeds for other acts of goodness.
I hope I'll get to see what these seeds have sown.

When I go to heaven,
Those will be the seeds that will produce the flowers
That we don't get to see in this world,
The flowers that only grow in heaven.

At once practical and visionary, the woman's narrative portrays flowers as generative symbols of kindness and compassion, love and grace. Not surprisingly, these themes resonate strongly with Thérèse's writings. When reminding her sister Pauline of a small notebook that the latter had given as a devotional tool prior to Thérèse's receiving First Holy Communion, Thérèse described how the journal became a kind of living sanctuary that

> aided me in preparing my heart through a sustained and thorough method. Although I had already prepared it for a long time, my heart needed a new thrust; it had to be filled with *fresh flowers* so that Jesus could rest there with pleasure. Every day I made a large number of fervent acts which made up so many *flowers*, and I offered up an even greater number of aspirations which you had written in my little book for every day, and these acts of love formed *flower buds*.[16]

Touching at the Edge: The Doubling of Life and Death

In Thérèse's writings and in end-of-life narratives, flowers often appear as symbols of love and of intimate proximity. These themes arose again as I met a woman who had been admitted to the Unit the previous day for pain management and for complications resulting from a leaking gastric tube. As the delivery of medical care unfolded all around her, I sat at the bedside and asked the woman if there was an image in her mind of something that held special meaning for her. Speaking softly but unhesitatingly, she described an intimate scene that I transcribed into a poetic artwork:

> *Touching at the Edge*
>
> *I got this picture the other night.*
> *It's of family, and it makes me feel good.*
> *It's of my family's hands.*
> *It's all of us.*
> *I liked the picture,*
> *And I wanted to keep it.*
>
> *In my family,*
> *We have all different ages.*
> *Because there were too many hands to put*
> *One on top of the other,*
> *Our hands are all kind of*
> *Touching at the edge.*

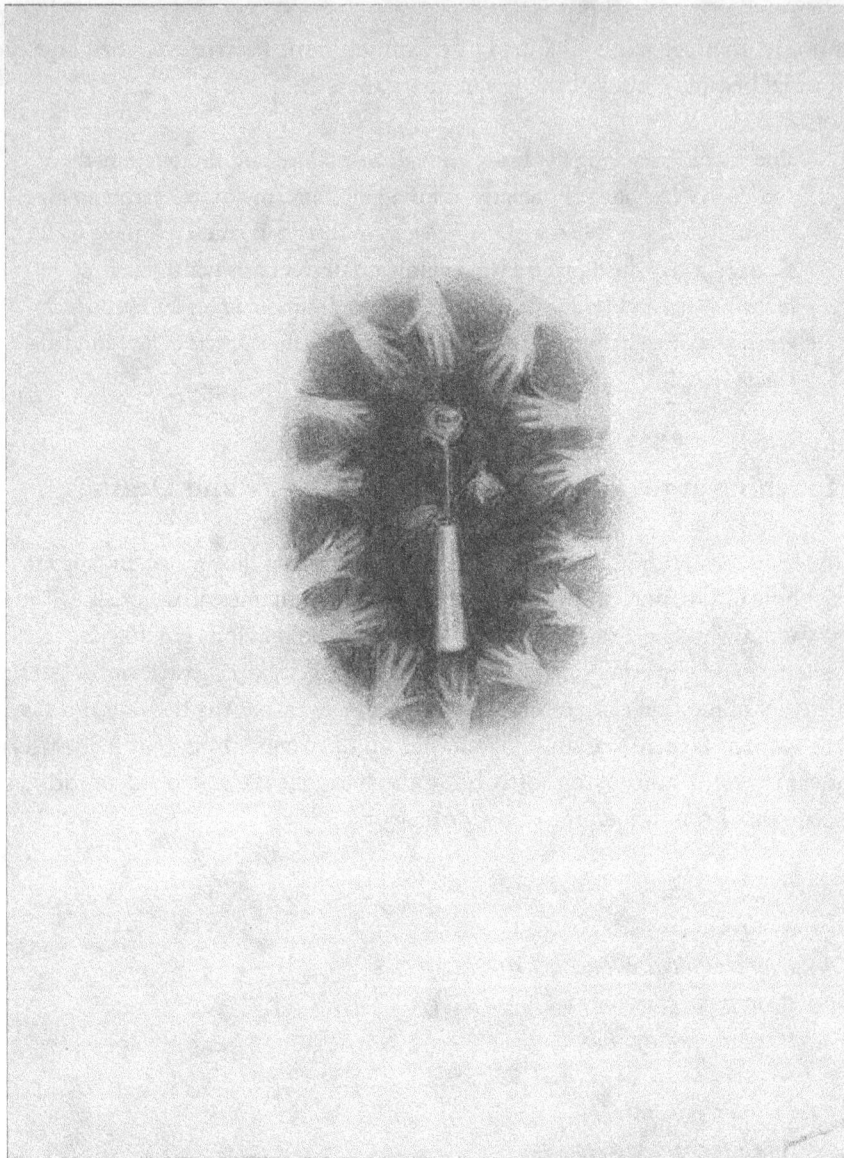

Figure 19: Lyn Smallwood, *Touching at the Edge*, 2021, graphite on white Strathmore drawing paper

As I read the story aloud, the woman cried softly and expressed her thanks. She then showed me the photograph of her family's clustered hands, and I realized that I was looking at a paradox—an image of the fullness of emptiness. As people's hands formed an open circle, each person's fingers nearly touched the fingers of the person next to them, and their hands created a constellation of presences. As I looked up from the picture on the woman's phone, I noticed a slender white budvase perched on the windowsill. The vase contained two yellow roses. One rose was opening beautifully on its upright stem, while the other was already drooping and faded. Despite their differences, the flowers were two of a kind and they clearly belonged together.

Lyn Smallwood's illustration, *Touching at the Edge* (Figure 19), presents a nested image in which various presences touch and support one another. The outer edges of the oval drawing display outspread fingers that form a ring of hands. A tall white budvase holding two long-stemmed roses sits at the center. While one flower opens, the other bud is limp and wilting. Both the circle of hands and the adjacent roses evoke a poignant sense of contingency, just as they convey the power and the fragility of life itself.

As I looked around the woman's room and took in these sights, I knew that, once again, I was standing in the presence of a rose from two gardens.

Notes

1. The imagery of pulling the weeds from the flowers also resonates with two bibli-
    cal parables, the Parable of the Sower (Matthew 13: 1–23), and the Parable of
    the Wheat and the Tares (Matthew 13: 24-42). Such parables are teaching sto-
    ries that draw on familiar organic and agricultural images as descriptive vehicles
    for conveying spiritual insights on cultivation and care.
2. In her related discussion of "Consecrating the Ordinary," the physician Rachel
    Naomi Remen comments on the ways in which sacred themes can be perceived
    in daily rituals and ordinary objects, much as she experienced in her garden. See
    Rachel Naomi Remen, *Kitchen Table Wisdom: Stories that Heal* (New York: Riv-
    erhead Books, 1996), 282–84.
3. Thomas R. Nevin contrasts the identity that Thérèse adopted as a warrior and
    a willing sacrificial victim of God's love with her self-construction as a child
    who gathers flowers for devotional offerings and who casts their petals at the
    throne of heaven. Nevin characterizes the latter as "trivial" and "playful" gestures
    that evoke both "the helpless child of the church" and the mythical "eternal
    feminine in its inviolate adolescence," which represents "an emblem of fertility
    and bounty." He further reads these typological identities in dialectical terms as
    "the Church Triumphant passing on her petals to the Church Militant." These
    conversant typologies are thus characterized as representing the "two-sidedness"
    of "a singular mission [of] suffering and playing." See Nevin, *Thérèse of Lisieux*,
    195–98. In contrast to this dialectical reading, I approach Thérèse's multifaceted
    engagement with floral imagery as expressing a sense of nonduality that can si-
    multaneously accommodate oppositional states of being.
4. Quoted in *Story of a Soul*, 74.
5. Quoted in *Story of a Soul*, 14.
6. Quoted in *Story of a Soul*, 14.
7. Regarding the significance of garden themes for people at the end of life, in his
    discussion of "Illness unto Death," Dr. Arthur Kleinman reproduces portions
    of a conversation between a doctor and a man who will soon succumb to meta-
    static colorectal cancer. Having made the choice to die at home, the man com-
    mented on the significance of his garden: "The garden—even till now I thought
    of a garden as something you look out into in order to escape the solipsism of
    yourself: Things moved and you saw them ... But now I think of my garden as a
    setting into which you project your feelings in order to organize them. You order

what is inside by looking in an outer, ordered space." At the very end of life, the man thus recognized the ways in which his garden served as a self-reflective tool, as an intermediate space that bridged his inner feelings and the landscape of the outer world, and vice versa. See Arthur Kleinman, *The Illness Narratives: Suffering, Healing, and the Human Condition* (New York: Basic Books, 1988), 147.

8. Quoted in *Story of a Soul*, 90–91.

9. Quoted in *Story of a Soul*, 37.

10. Quoted in *St. Thérèse of Lisieux*, 48.

11. Quoted in *St. Thérèse of Lisieux*, 239.

12. Quoted in *St. Thérèse of Lisieux*, 62.

13. Quoted in Thurston and Attwater, *Butler's Lives of the Saints*, vol. 4, 15.

14. Quoted in *St. Thérèse of Lisieux*, 256.

15. Quoted in *Story of a Soul*, 267–68.

16. Quoted in *Story of a Soul*, 73–74.

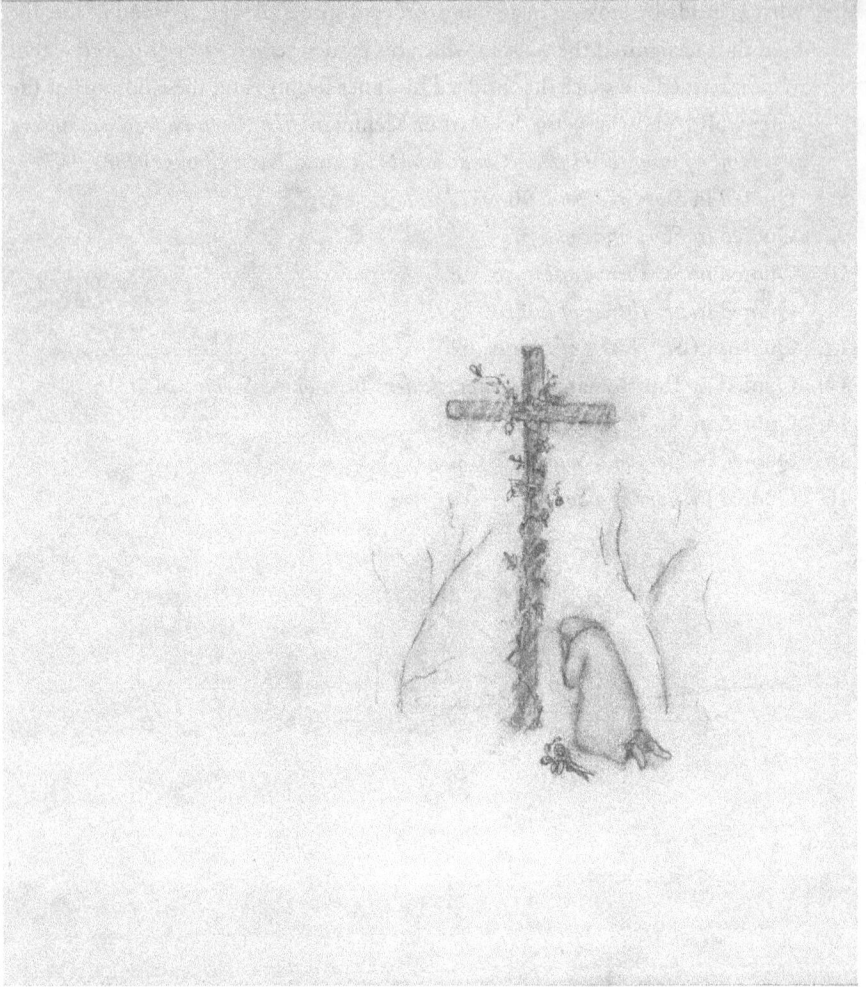

Figure 20: Lyn Smallwood, *I've Always Loved Crosses*, 2020, graphite on white Strathmore drawing paper

Chapter Five

The Cross and the Crown of Thorns: Sacrifice, Suffering, and Consolation

I've Always Loved Crosses: The Strength of Faith

Even though the woman had never heard of Thérèse of Lisieux, her narrative resonated strongly with the imagery of this saint. The woman described herself as Christian but not Catholic, and she told me how

I've Always Loved Crosses

My image now would definitely be of a cross.
This image has been with me for the past few years,
And it relates to things I was going through.
But, I've always loved crosses.

This particular cross has roses coming down from it,
And it has a figure at the bottom, kneeling.
This figure is me,
At the base,
And the roses are red.

Like the woman's story, Lyn Smallwood's illustration, *I've Always Loved Crosses* (Figure 20), is elegant, minimal, and deeply evocative. The drawing's shaded pencil lines soften the otherwise prominent geometric forms within this focused composition. In this image, a woman kneels at the base of a cross, over which grows a vine of climbing roses. The cross appears at once as a sacred symbol and as a kind of garden trellis. On the ground, a small bouquet of roses lays at the woman's side; both the flowers and the prayers serve as devotional offerings. By engaging this imagery, the artwork expresses the ways in which some of the most beautiful things and some of the most difficult things can appear as coextensive presences. This paradox can become especially intense as people face pronounced suffering and they begin to reimagine themselves at the end of life.

In this chapter, I examine some of the ways in which individuals engage the imagery of the cross as a source of strength, consolation, and spiritual power when facing end-of-life transitions. Within Christian iconography in general, and in end-of-life narratives in particular, the cross represents a consummate signifier of ultimate things, including interwoven conceptions of faith and devotion, sacrifice and salvation.[1] These themes also appear as leitmotifs in the writings of Thérèse of Lisieux, who is traditionally depicted as carrying a cross draped with roses. Just as the biblical story of the crucifixion is associated with conceptions of forgiveness and redemption, these subjects can provide people with vital sources of solace and inspiration by affirming the presence of ongoing life.

Yet at the outset, I will emphasize that *in no way am I advocating the glamorization, romanticization, or even, the particular value of any image or practice that is based in a personal or religious identification with issues of trauma, pain, or suffering.* This includes, but is not limited to, substitutive or redemptive suffering—that is, of an individual's willingly assuming pain as an act of personal atonement or as an offering made on behalf of another.[2] Both in life and at the end of life, religion can represent a highly ambivalent coping mechanism. In this chapter, I provide examples of both positive and negative religious coping strategies.

Slapping God in the Face: Judgment, Fear, and Alienation

The end of life can be a particularly fraught time, as individuals and families attempt to negotiate an interwoven set of personal beliefs, shared pains, and collective fears. In these difficult circumstances, some people will adopt a rigid approach to their religious beliefs and practices. Even as they emphatically profess their faith, some individuals will still see death as a state of judgment, punishment, or the nothingness of complete annihilation. These themes can appear symbolically as people's crosses to bear.

To illustrate these complex subjects, I will share three stories that exemplify negative religious coping strategies, in which people engage the shadow sides of spirituality. The first story is entitled *An Impeccable Posture and the Letter of the Law*. One day I met an elderly man who had spent his entire professional career as a lawyer, and later, as a judge. Now he faced the end of life from advanced lymphoma. The nurses told me that, when he's awake, he "holds court" in his room, and he can be quite demanding. I witnessed some of these qualities firsthand when I entered the room and saw the man literally giving a blessing to a younger family member. After he had finished, I introduced myself and chatted with the patient and his soft-spoken wife. Ultimately, their voices converged to form an artwork. The man characterized his wife as exemplifying "a perfect approach to life." When I asked what that meant for him, he replied, "She has an impeccable posture. I have never known of her doing a single bad thing in her life. Never a violation of the scripture, Old or New Testament. I have been led by her example." Together we created a poetic narrative that focused on the man's life, and which concluded with his powerful affirmation of religious faith:

Through Life to Death to Life

My image is to have a relationship with God,
And to pass quickly into His care and love.
God will be with me in my passing:
Through life to death to life.

After I read the words aloud, the man cried and he expressed his concern that he may not get into heaven because the standards of God could be greater than human ones, and he may not measure up. The man also confessed his fear of being separated from his beloved wife of so many decades. At the end of life, religion represented an ambivalent source of both comfort and distress, as the man voiced his deep concerns regarding issues of mercy and judgment, faith and fear, and his ultimate inability to know or control the outcome. This story exemplifies the place where the letter of the law meets the unwritten words of the kingdom of heaven. Concerned that he may not have met the highest standards or maintained the most stringent regimens, the judge became apprehensive as he anticipated a continuation of judgment, yet one that he now faced from the other side of the bench. Thus he turned to Christian scripture to discern "the letter of the law," just as he faced a situation that inherently exceeded the boundaries of language and knowledge.

    Similar themes arose in a related story that I will call *How Is This Helping?* On another day, I met a family who drew on Christian scripture in what I can only describe as a kind of terror management strategy. This fearful response came not from the patient herself, but from a close family member. The patient's husband, sister, and elderly mother were gathered at the bedside, and the woman's sister had been reading the Bible aloud. When she finished a particular verse, I introduced myself and briefly described the creative work. Before the patient could speak, her sister demanded, "What is the purpose of all this? We have our image of Jesus, so why would we need any other image?" The patient's elderly mother then intervened, saying that the question was for her other daughter to answer. The woman lying in the bed quietly stated:

> *My image is of God and family.*
> *God is with me.*
> *God is love.*

When I invited the woman to expand on her image of God and family, her sister foreclosed the conversation by aggressively asserting: "That is in scripture!" The patient was clearly hesitant to respond further, as if she feared provoking a negative reaction from her family. I quickly saw that this encounter was emotionally exhausting for the woman, so I inscribed her brief phrases into a handmade paper journal, and I thanked everyone and prepared to leave. As I turned toward the door, the patient's sister indignantly asked, "How is this helping? This should be all about worship!"

Much as in *An Impeccable Posture and the Letter of the Law, How Is This Helping?* tells a story of fear and suffering, in which people try to control an inherently uncontrollable situation. These stories feature a sense of religious literalism—that is, of rigid adherence to scripture, or to the letter of the law. While reading biblical passages aloud may well have comforted and united the family, it also had the chilling effect of foreclosing individual speech and presence. The result was that, at the end of life, a woman's unique voice became eclipsed by the orthodox voice of scripture.

Another complex example of negative religious coping arose as a woman described her fear of *Slapping God in the Face.* This attractive middle-aged woman told me that, in her life she had "delved into God," but she also feared that she had "slapped God in the face." The woman was a new transfer to the Palliative Care Unit, and the medical team had characterized her as high-distress. While describing the difficult situations that she and her family faced, the woman was clearly filled with rage and fear. We spent a considerable amount of time talking together, and after a little while, the woman began telling me wonderful things about her children and grandchildren. These statements formed the basis of her artwork. The woman then started speaking more broadly about her religious and spiritual life, and she described a personal experience so powerful that it literally left her shaking in awe. Now facing the end of her life, the woman could not fully reconcile this event with her traditional religious life, and this created great inner conflict. As she told me:

I've had experiences with God
That some people wouldn't understand.
I'm Pentecostal.
There was one time we were having a ladies' prayer meeting,
And I delved into God.

I'm in there praying,
And you could feel something in there.
Something was happening,
But you didn't know what.
We're praying, and holding hands,
And some of the women are speaking in tongues.
You know you're supposed to do something,
But you don't know what.
The lady leading the meeting said,
"Just do what God tells you."

She got the preacher,
And he said, "You need to step out and give yourself to God."
I was scared, and I was shaking,
With what I felt in that power.
I felt warmth, I felt love, and I felt peace.
I felt the power of His presence.

Not surprisingly, the intensity of this experience stayed with the woman, and the memory returned to her at the end of her life. Yet after I read her words aloud, the woman shared her fear that she might be going to hell because she did not allow herself to let go completely and speak in tongues when she felt God's presence in the prayer group. Because of her inability to surrender fully, she felt that she had "slapped God in the face" and that she had "refused Him by being scared and not speaking up and allowing Him to come forward." I reminded her of the positive aspects of the experience, particularly the sense of love, warmth, and peace that had moved her so greatly. She then admitted that she did not fully trust me, and she began to question me about my own spiritual beliefs. Because I did not belong to the Pentecostal Church, the woman remained uncertain about our encounter. At the end of the visit, she told me, "I think maybe God sent you to me." But then she expressed her concern that "maybe the devil has sent you." Given the woman's high levels of emotional and spiritual distress, after the visit I spoke with the other members of the palliative care team, and both the attending physician and the chaplain promised to follow up shortly. To this day I continue to think about this woman, and I hope that she was ultimately able to return to that place of peace, warmth, and love.

He Reserved a Great Number of Crosses For Me: Thérèse's Varying Perspectives on the Cross

Like many people at the end of life, Thérèse expressed a complex engagement with the symbol of the cross. In *Story of a Soul* she recalled how, as a child, she made "a spectacle" of herself by wearing "a big crucifix" that her sister had given her, and how, in her youth, she felt "a *great desire* to suffer, and at the same time, the interior assurance that Jesus reserved a great number of crosses for me."[3] Repeating the prayers that she was taught, Thérèse related how she felt a sense of attraction to suffering as a means to imitate an example of love, although admittedly, she did not understand this phenomenon well. As a young girl, Thérèse was surrounded by Christian devotional imagery. After experiencing the death of her mother and the loss of two of her beloved older sisters to the cloistered Carmel, Thérèse spent extended time in the attic of the family home, which contained a bookstand with flowers, candles, and a statue of the Blessed Virgin. On the far end of the wall hung a large cross fashioned out of black wood.[4]

Later in life, Thérèse adopted a complex perspective on the cross. At the end of her life, Thérèse's older sister Pauline recorded how Thérèse "told me how she'd worn her little iron cross for a long time and that it had made her sick. She told me, too, that it wasn't God's will for her, nor for us to throw ourselves into great mortifications; this sickness was proof of it." Pauline also recorded how Thérèse advised her fellow nuns: "Don't be troubled, little sisters, if I suffer very much and if you see in me, as I've already said, no sign of happiness at the moment of my death. Our Lord really died as a Victim of Love, and you see what His agony was! ... All this says nothing." Pauline also reminded Thérèse of her prayers in which she expressed a desire for suffering, to which

Thérèse responded: "I wanted to suffer and I've been heard. I have suffered very much for several days now. One morning, during my act of thanksgiving after Communion, I felt the agonies of death … and with it no consolation!" As she lay dying, Thérèse was handed a crucifix, which she kissed tenderly. As she did so, Pauline recorded Thérèse as saying: "He is dead! I prefer when they represent Him as dead, because then I think He is no longer suffering."[5] Even as she faced the end of her own life, Thérèse felt great compassion for the suffering of Christ in all of his humanity.

We Collect Crosses: Affirming Family Bonds Through the Cross

People at the end of life will similarly express an intimate connection with the figure of Christ, and the cross will often appear as an image of comfort and continuity. One young woman woke up just long enough to tell me what it means to have

My Mom's Wooden Rosary

My Mom's wooden rosary hangs
Over the head of my hospital bed.
We grew up Catholic.
It gives me security to have this religious life.
Mom puts the rosary in my hands when I'm asleep.
It gives me a feeling of security,
Of going in God's will.

For this young woman, the cross provided a tangible source of comfort and accompaniment, of presence and faith that further strengthened the love of the family during a period of shattering pain. On another afternoon I visited with an extremely close, middle-aged couple. The man could barely speak due to his advanced tongue cancer. Yet his wife still understood him perfectly, and she was able to communicate for both of them. When I asked about their images, the woman told me: "We collect crosses," which they saw as "symbols of peace and salvation." Over many years, they had received gifts of iron, wooden, and ceramic crosses, all of which were displayed in a colorful collage on their living room wall. The wife then spoke of her family's rootedness in their Christian faith, and how they felt they were "living the cross." For this family, the cross

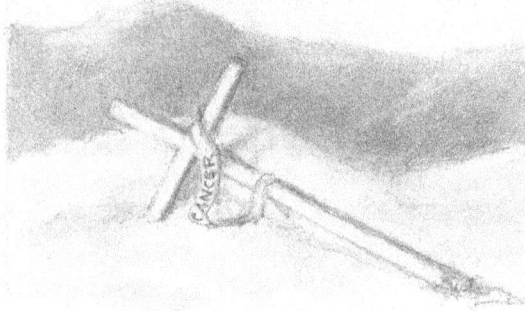

Figure 21: Lyn Smallwood, *The Cross With "Cancer": He's Never Lost His Faith*, 2015, graphite on white Arches paper

represented a shared symbol of strength, unity, and consolation during a time of trial:

We Collect Crosses

We collect crosses.
My family is very spiritual.
We have found through this experience
That we have been able to endure
More than we thought we could.
It has strengthened us
As a family.

He's Never Lost His Faith

When I first entered the room, the young woman in bed was deeply asleep, with her eyes rolled back in her head. Her devoted father sat in a chair at her bedside, and the woman awoke when she heard us talking. As she and I visited together, her father took the opportunity to step out and get some air. I learned that the woman was one of several children in a large Catholic family, and that they had lost their mother to cancer when she was still very young. Now the woman was sad because her father "has to live through that again." At the end of the visit, she told me that I provided an important service, and I told her that I was honored to be with her and her family at this time. I then suggested that the woman dedicate the artwork to her father, an idea that she readily embraced.

The Cross With "Cancer": He's Never Lost His Faith

My image is of a cross
With the word "cancer" written on it.
The letters are written on a banner
That is white and gold,
And the cross is laying on its side.

For me, this image is my way out.
It's what's going to take me,
But the whole time,

I know God will be with me.
I feel sad because I'm leaving my family,
But happy, because I'm going to heaven.

My dad is responsible for my faith.
He's done a lot of things in the church.
My mom died when she was young,
And my dad did everything for us.
Everything is wonderful about my dad.
He's so humble, and he always thinks he has to do more for us.
But everything he's done is more than enough.

This image is for him,
Because it's the most special thing I can do.
He's never lost his faith,
And I don't think he ever will.

The cancer will take me out of this world,
But never out of his life.

Lyn Smallwood's drawing, *The Cross With "Cancer": He's Never Lost His Faith* (Figure 21), depicts a cross lying on its side in a remote, hilly landscape. The word "Cancer" appears on a ribbon that is draped softly over the cross's horizontal frame. In contrast to the rigid geometric lines of the archetypal wooden form, the rolling mountains in the background create a continuous silhouette that modulates and softens the scene. In a landscape that is devoid of all human forms, the placement of the cross on this elevated ground makes this spare image monumental—a symbol of presence and of transcendence.

When I returned to the hospital the following week, I saw the woman briefly, as she was being wheeled back to her room following a CT scan. At that point she had lost the functional use of her limbs. I leaned over the bed to say hello, but it wasn't clear if she recognized me. Her affect was flat and detached, and she appeared to be very withdrawn. Clearly, the woman was pulling deep into herself as she prepared to make her journey. This made me especially grateful that we had the opportunity to visit the previous week and produce an artwork that reflected what mattered most to her, both in life and at the end of her life.

The Crown of Thorns: Images of Sacrifice and Devotion

People's images of the cross can be particularly striking when they are accompanied by ribbons or flowers, symbols of sacrifice and devotion. As we have seen, Thérèse associated flowers with practical acts of care, with the "little things" she did out of love. As she acknowledged, "I am the smallest of creatures; I know my misery and my feebleness, but I know also how much noble and generous hearts love to do good."[6] As she imagined love being translated into acts of kindness, she vowed to "strew flowers" as offerings to God:

> I have no other means of proving my love for You other than that of strewing flowers, that is, not allowing one little sacrifice to escape, not one look, one word, profiting by all the smallest things and doing them through love. I desire to suffer for love and even to rejoice through love; and in this way I shall strew flowers before Your throne. I shall not come upon one without *unpetalling* it for You. While I am strewing my flowers, I shall sing, for could one cry while doing such a joyous action? I shall sing even when I must gather my flowers in the midst of thorns, and my song will be all the more melodious in proportion to the length and sharpness of the thorns.[7]

Through such floral imagery, Thérèse forged connections between pain and joy, between human vulnerability and numinous divinity. These themes become particularly evident in Thérèse's engagement with the Holy Face. As a discalced Carmelite nun, Thérèse assumed the double name of Thérèse of the Child Jesus and the Holy Face, the latter signifying her devotion to Jesus throughout the extreme trials of suffering associated with the crucifixion.[8] Before she entered the Carmel, Thérèse and her family became members of the Archconfraternity of Reparation to the Holy Face at Tours, a group that advocated prayers of devotion to the Holy Face as expressions of redemptive suffering.[9] In *Story of a Soul* Thérèse observed that "The little flower transplanted to Mt. Carmel was to expand under the shadow of the cross. The tears and blood of Jesus were to be her dew, and her Sun was His adorable Face veiled with tears. Until my coming to Carmel, I had never fathomed the depths of the treasures hidden in the Holy Face."[10] Thérèse described meditating on the face of Jesus and offering her love and compassion amidst the agony of his suffering. Such experiences enabled her to recognize the beauty of divine presence embedded within the disfiguration that marked extreme states of human suffering. As Thérèse engaged in a devotional practice that both incorporated, and lay beyond, established categorical distinctions between ugliness and beauty, tears

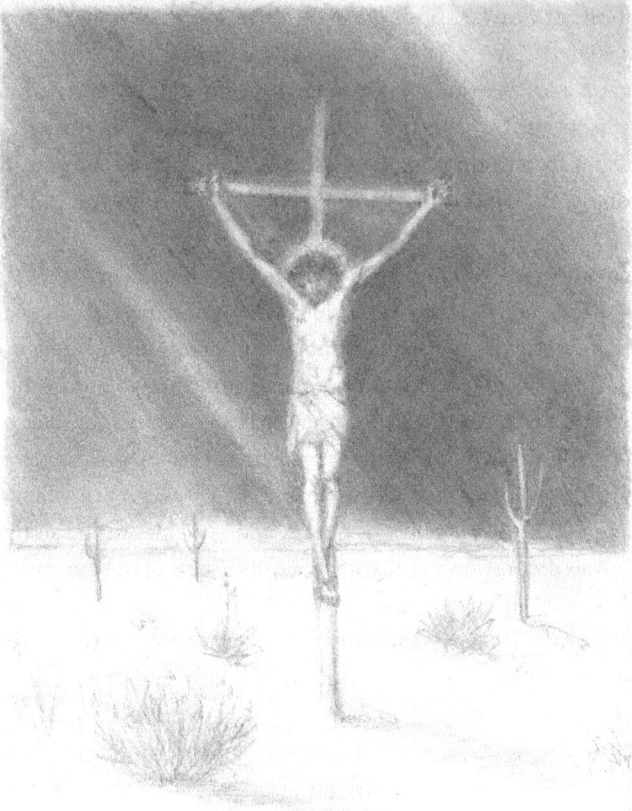

Figure 22: Lyn Smallwood, *The Crown of Thorns*, 2015, graphite on white Arches paper

and blood became transformed into sun and treasure.[11] Through this devotion, Thérèse was able to see beauty when there was nothing left to see.

The Crown of Thorns

One day I met an older man whose end-of-life imagery engaged the crown of thorns. The man had just completed his first hospice consult, and I was a bit surprised that he wanted to work together because his affect was so flat. I asked him where he was from, and the man told me about his home in the Sonoran desert of Arizona. He emphasized that he "is not super-religious," yet his imagery represented a striking expression of faith. The man's tone was very terse, yet he spoke eloquently on what he saw as the ultimate sacrificial offering:

The Crown Of Thorns

My image now is just the cross.
I've been thinking about it a lot lately.
I'm trying to be Christian.

I love flowers.
I like the cactus and century plants,
The plants of the Western outdoors.
That's what grows well up where I live.
You don't have to tend to them.
They take care of themselves.

Cacti have thorns.
On the cross,
Christ had a crown of thorns,
And it was bleeding.

The man's narrative fuses familiar Christian reference points with the distinctive ambiance of the desert Southwest. Lyn Smallwood translates this hybrid imagery into *The Crown of Thorns* (Figure 22). This soft pencil drawing features a Western-style version of the traditional crucifixion scene as the figure of Christ appears in a spare desert landscape filled with century plants and saguaro cacti. Resonating with the plants' spiky leaves, a crown of thorns is perched on Christ's bleeding brow, beneath a brightly glowing halo. In an otherwise darkened scene, rays of light illuminate this stark vision of a cross in the desert.

During times of intense suffering and vulnerability, crucifixion images can help people to visualize the humanity of the sacred, and to connect the sacred to their own human lives. One lovely woman described herself as a devout Baptist, and she shared her composite image of

The Wooden Cross, the Crown of Thorns, and Eternal Life

My image is of Jesus dying on the cross.
I see the wooden cross, and the crown of thorns on His head.
And I see all the suffering He did,
And the hurt and the pain that He went through for us.

He went through all of this for me,
And I know He's going to be there for me,
In my pain.
He toted that cross to give me eternal life.
It's just a blessing,
And I can't thank Him enough,
Or God, for sending His son to do this,
For me, and for all of us.

The Good Lord is still blessing me every day.
It's His plan, and I have to live whatever His plan is,
In His time.
I just thank Him,
That He gave me another day
To see my family
And to live in this beautiful world
That He created.

As the woman produced an artwork that reads like a prayer, she drew on the imagery of the cross and the crown of thorns to voice her gratitude for divine accompaniment, and her faith in the promise of eternal life. People at the end of life will often express such a personal connection with the figure of the crucified Christ as they identify with the experience of extreme suffering, and they affirm a sense of devotion. One day I met an older woman who was originally from Viet Nam. She described a mystical connection with the crucified Christ and the bond of suffering and trust which, she felt, they shared deeply:

In Life, and in Death

My image is of the cross.
I would be like one person at the foot of the cross.
And, I would be looking at it.
I see this in meditation.
I meditate every day.
The picture is of the Lord on the cross,
And He's not dead.
He's looking down, looking at me,
And we keep talking in prayer.
He says that He bore everything for me.
I don't have to give anything to get His favor.
I'm just taking it in.
I just receive.

I was restless, and anxious, and worrying.
This gives me a sense of rest.
Even though I know the situation is tough,
In the meantime, I can just rest.
I trust in Him,
In life, and in death.

The woman prayed and cried as we worked together. Despite her suffering, her eyes were filled with light and grace. While such crucifixion imagery can be extremely difficult to contemplate, it also proved to be instrumental in comforting the woman as she visualized the humanity of divinity.

Because of My Faith: Witnessing Suffering and Cultivating Strategies of Presence

Just as the cross represents an iconic image of suffering and devotion, people at the end of life will often couple associations of trauma and pain with a corresponding sense of hope and uplift. One day I visited with a young woman who described the difficult life she had experienced, including her earlier battle with drug abuse, and her current struggle with advanced intestinal cancer.

While she told a story of serial hardships, she also described how she was sustained

Because of My Faith

My image is of something Christian—
A cross.
This is because of my faith.
I have a strong faith in Jesus.
And He's what keeps me going.
I see Him with brown sandals, and a white gown,
And as a bright light.
This image makes me feel happy and contented.
It brings peace of mind.

In the last few years
This has become more important to me.
I became Christian,
And then I was diagnosed with cancer.
I was bitter at first.
And then, I was free of cancer for a while.
I was in remission.
And I regained my faith.
But then, when the cancer came back,
I didn't give up my faith this time.
And that makes me feel strong.

After I read the story aloud, both the woman and I felt a palpable shift in the atmosphere of the room. She cried as I sat holding her hand. Now facing the end of her life, the woman associated her Christian faith with both her frailty and her strength.

Another powerful story of doubt and faith arose as I visited with a middle-aged man. The medical team told me that he suffered from "a terrible sarcoma." His pain was extremely difficult to control, and heavy doses of medication were making him sleepy. Yet the man woke up when I entered the room. He immediately told me that his Christian faith was an important part of his life, and that it had been tested severely in the past few weeks. Amidst this crucible of pain and doubt, the man affirmed his faith in divine presence:

That Proven Strength: I Know He's There

The image of Jesus on the cross
Is the image that lets me know—
And believe—
That He did this for me.
I've had a joyful life,
And I know that I've had that life
Because of His dying on the cross.

I was devout from my youth until a few weeks ago.
Then, I was in total misery.
I still believed all these things,
But it seems like that proven strength
Jumped around a bit.

I haven't gone through anything like
What He's gone through.
And, He's with me now.
Oh, yes.
I just know.
I don't know how I know.
But, I can feel His presence.
I know He's there.
Even though I've been in complete torture for the past few weeks,
My belief is there,
And my faith is still there.
And now, listening to myself talk,
I think this is helping me
To know that He's there.

When I first entered the room, the man was shaking in pain. Yet as we spoke together, he visibly relaxed. His pain was still present, but he was more alert and at ease. When I read his words aloud, both he and his wife cried in gratitude. In this extremely difficult situation, the man's words provided a means to recognize his connection to the sacred, and this sense of recognition allowed him to be present to himself during a difficult period of transition.

After shadowing me on a similar visit on the Palliative Care Unit, a pre-medical student shared her perception that such end-of-life narratives allow patients to recognize their own monumental strength and beauty, both in spite of and within their experiences of suffering. She further observed that, by expressing these themes, the artworks can redefine the possibilities of life for people who are still living.[12] These comments have helped me to recognize the ways in which the work of the Artist In Residence can help to negotiate the extremely complex relations between trauma and presence, both for the person and for those around them, just as the visits can produce images of transcendence that lie both within and beyond the familiar boundaries of life itself.

The Three Crosses: I'm Seeing Them Now: Visionary Presence at the End of Life

Sometimes these sacred images lend themselves to expressions of visionary consciousness. When this occurs, there can be a sense that a person is inhabiting multiple domains at once. This was the case the day that a middle-aged man shared his end-of-life vision of

The Three Crosses

My image is of the three crosses,
And the middle cross has blood flowing from it.
It is my image.
It is my vision.

That is the power of the blood of Jesus.
Nothing else can do the job
Except the blood of Jesus.

Actually, there is an expansion of this image.
Behind Jesus is the Holy Spirit,
And then, God the Father.

This image originally came to me over forty years ago.
And then, it came on and off during my life,
Up until the moment that you came in today.

I see this image,
And I feel very blessed.

And, I'm seeing it now.

In such complex imagery, the presence of the suffering and dying body become invested with spiritual associations in ways that bind the physical and the metaphysical registers evermore closely.[13] In grounding such conceptions of the sacred within the framework of human experience, the artworks appear as vehicles that allow the spiritual to become even more fully immersed in the existential concerns of humanity.

Connecting Worlds: The Cross Lies at the Axes of Separation and Conjunction

In end-of-life narratives, the cross can appear as an ambivalent symbol of suffering and devotion that links the human and the divine realms through the imagery of life and death. Just as the cross is associated with the descent of sacred presence into the vulnerable interstices of human life, so too is it associated with the ascent of humanity. When viewed structurally, the cross is a dialogical form that arises at the conjunction of two intersecting axes. The cross's vertical axis is upright and hierarchical, extending from the base of the earth to the heavenly domain. This vertical axis serves at once as a pathway of ascent and descent, and by incorporating the two poles, it transcends the distance between them. Similarly, the cross's horizontal axis can be seen as reflecting the expansiveness of life itself. Just as this axis extends laterally, it appears as a level pathway that encompasses all things.

Thérèse's writings can also be seen as unfolding at the conjunction of the horizontal and the vertical axes, as though poised in the place where the frailty, humility, and humanity of the little way meet the expansive grandeur of the sacred.[14] Rather than presenting an impossible distance between the human and the divine realms, Thérèse's writings and end-of-life narratives repeatedly emphasize their conjunction. In so doing, the divine seemingly becomes accessible through an intimate form of mystical humanism. Throughout the images, the cross appears as a nondual symbol that incorporates the existential and the spiritual, the base and the exalted, the finite and the infinite. This formulation merges the bitter and the sweet (or, in Thérèse's terms, the vinegar and the sugar), while encompassing ugliness and beauty, death and life itself. As these seemingly opposite subjects coalesce, they appear as the one that are two *and* the two that are one—and thus, as a rose from two gardens.

Notes

1. These themes resonate with the deep roots of the hospice movement. Dame Cicely Saunders, the founder of the modern hospice movement, drew on her Christian faith as she formulated a pioneering approach to the treatment of composite pain, a construct that included spiritual as well as physical pain. As Saunders observed of her own clinical work: "We meet some who seem to have had little chance of a worthwhile life or death and find that our belief in a God who has himself gone through the rejection and death of a world of random pain and catastrophe keeps us close to such people with trust and hope for them." See Cicely Saunders, Mary Baines, and Robert Dunlop, *Living With Dying: A Guide to Palliative Care*, 3rd ed. (New York: Oxford University Press, 1995), 55. Saunders's approach to care thus extended to both the body and the spirit, and she advocated a practice that emphasized the values of forgiveness and acceptance, faith and trust, meaning and peace, and belief in something greater than oneself. While Saunders ultimately asserted the value of freedom and openness when responding to another person's spiritual pain, Michael Wright and David Clark have noted that, in Saunders's approach, "Attitudes toward human suffering provide a key to understanding the religious dimensions of a good death. For the Christian, for example, suffering may be regarded as a means of transformation, linked somehow to the suffering and redemptive mission of Jesus." See Michael Wright and David Clark, "Cicely Saunders and the Development of Hospice Palliative Care," *Religious Understandings of a Good Death in Hospice Palliative Care*, ed. Harold Coward and Kelli I. Stajduhar (Albany: SUNY Press, 2012), 17–18.

2. For a critical reading of Thérèse's childhood exposure to substitutive suffering, see Furlong, *Thérèse of Lisieux*, 56–57.

3. Quoted in *Story of a Soul*, 76, 79.

4. See *Story of a Soul*, 90.

5. Quoted in *St. Thérèse of Lisieux*, 115, 56, 154.

6. Quoted in *Story of a Soul*, 195–96.

7. Quoted in *Story of a Soul*, 196–97.

8. Photographs of Thérèse taken at the Carmel show her holding an iconic image of the child Jesus in one hand, and in the other, an equally well-known drawing of Jesus during the crucifixion, with lowered eyes and flowing tears. Such popular cultural imagery was prominent in Thérèse's historical context.

9. The devotion of reparation to the Holy Face of Jesus is a practice that the Carmelite nun, Sister Mary of St. Peter, first expressed in mid-nineteenth-century France. The purpose of this offering is to make reparations for sins offending God. This devotion was officially recognized by Pope Leo XIII in 1885. Regarding these practices, see https://theholyface.com/prayers-of-the-holy-face/.

10. As Thérèse affirmed in her prayer to the Holy Face of Jesus: "Under those disfigured features, I recognize Thy infinite Love and I am consumed with the desire to love Thee and make Thee loved by all men." Quoted in *Story of a Soul*, 151–52.

11. On these themes, see also Thérèse's poems "A Withered Rose" and "To Scatter Flowers" in *Poems of St. Teresa, Carmelite of Lisieux, known as the 'Little Flower of Jesus'* (Grand Rapids, MI: Christian Classics Ethereal Library, n.d.): http://www.ccel.org/download.html?url=/ccel/therese/poems.pdf.

12. I am grateful to Dr. Zoe Tao for sharing her observations on these subjects.

13. Regarding these subjects, Robert Orsi has noted the ways in which cultural constructions of the heaven world can serve as powerful compensatory mechanisms for human suffering: "The work that heaven does in culture seems as clear as the work that death does, if for the opposite reasons. Heaven grounds the realness of the otherwise contingent worlds that we humans make for ourselves in the face of the nothingness, chaos, and oblivion that are the facts of creaturely existence and the results of the actions and plans of men and women. Our short lives acquire not only purpose but also grandeur and drama when they are set against the horizon of sacred history." See Orsi, *History and Presence*, 204.

14. Peter-Thomas Rohrbach has similarly observed that Thérèse's life can be seen as unfolding on two planes at once, including the natural and the supernatural, the domains of humanity and of grace. See Rohrbach, *The Search for St. Thérèse*, 25.

Figure 23: Lyn Smallwood, *The Flickering Flame: We Find Our Way Back*, 2016, graphite on white Arches paper

Chapter Six

"Prayer Burns with the Fire of Love": Warriors, Faith, and the Courage of the Heart

A Burning, Flickering Flame

"He sleeps a lot, but when he's awake, he's delightful. So are his sister and his father. And, they all have stories."

The chaplain's description was brief but promising. I knocked lightly on the man's door in case he was asleep. Fortunately, the middle-aged man was wide awake, and he remained alert throughout the visit. His sister was by his side, and it was clear from their postures that the two siblings were very close. Perched along the window ledge were several statues of Catholic saints; their venerable presences transformed the edge of the windowsill into an informal devotional altar. As we visited, the man told a powerful story that interwove traditional religious subjects with insights drawn from his personal life:

The Flickering Flame: We Find Our Way Back

Right now, my image would be of a flame,
The outline of a cathedral,
And the silhouettes of my family.
My family is wonderful, dedicated, and very dear.
They just gleam with love,
And they have endless amounts of love to give.
When we were young,
We would go to a lake house.
We were surrounded by state park land,
And we learned something there

That we took with us in life.
We would go out and get lost in the woods,
And then we would find our way back.
That's childhood—and it's adulthood, too.
It was important then, and it's important now.

The church gives me a feeling of warmth,
And of family love.
Something that powerful is like a foundation.
My image is of an outline of a cathedral.
It looks antique, classical, and authentic.
My image is also of a burning, flickering flame.
I've always been passionate about flames.
I don't know why,
But for me, the flickering flame of a white candle
Has always been a symbol of purity, passion, and love.

We get caught up in life
And then, we find our way back.

When I returned to the hospital the following week, the man had slipped into a coma and he was actively dying. As I have witnessed on so many occasions, sometimes people will become intensely lucid in the final days or hours preceding their death. At this transitional juncture, a person's words and images, their gestures and facial expressions, can take on heightened meanings. In this case, the man's story reflects his pronounced sense of courage, clarity, and faith. The man had reached a place of peace and his imagery was at once intimate, sacred, and deeply radiant.

At the center of Lyn Smallwood's illustration (Figure 23) lies the flickering flame of a single slender white candle. This vertical form both illuminates and obscures the adjacent outlines of a cathedral with fluted columns and twin domed roofs topped with crosses. Much as in the man's story, these traditional architectural elements make the building look "antique, classical, and authentic." The cathedral is surrounded by a dark sky, which provides a sense of ambient contrast, just as it consolidates the drawing's focus on the central white void of the flame. As the scene recedes into the background, the view becomes progressively softer and more abstract. When the pictorial elements are taken together, the drawing evokes a sense that a man holding a brightly lit candle is about to approach the steps of a cathedral, a sacred space that he now longs to enter.

Just as *The Flickering Flame: We Find Our Way Back* relates a man's deep love for his family and their shared tradition of Roman Catholicism, this is a courageous story of origins and returns, of the candle and the flame that consumes it. While facing the end of life, these subjects provided the man with both a solid foundation and an etheric glow. As the historian of religion Robert Orsi has observed, such expressions of courage and confidence in the face of death represent traditional signs of moral strength in Catholicism, as the needs and the prayers of people become visible in the flames of the candles that fill Catholic devotional spaces.[1] Approaching these themes from a complementary perspective, the historian of religious visual culture David Morgan has commented on the capacity of words and images to "detach motifs from one cultural setting and transpose them to a new context to be re-enchanted as part of a new way of seeing or feeling." Something similar can occur at the end of life when, in Morgan's terms, people engage imagery that offers "a direct experience of selfhood when they have suffered the press of identity crisis."[2]

Much like Thérèse of Lisieux, people at the end of life will often tell powerful stories of bravery, faith, and courage. Throughout her life, Thérèse showed great strength in the wake of pronounced suffering. This was particularly the case when she faced her own premature death from tuberculosis at the age of twenty-four. While these are certainly not easy subjects, such expressions of courage and faith can become matters of vital importance. As individuals openly confront their imminent death, they often appear as sources of strength and inspiration to those around them.

She Was Thinking of Us: Courage at the End of Life

In her writings, Thérèse reflected on the ways in which her sense of connection to divine presence enabled the courageous acts that she was able to perform during her lifetime. As Thérèse noted, "God never refuses that first grace that gives one the courage to act; afterwards, the heart is strengthened and one advances from victory to victory."[3] At the end of her life, Thérèse shared a beautiful image of how such light radiates from one point to another. When describing her understanding of how the presence of a holy figure can endow a person with grace, Thérèse recalled how one of her fellow nuns

> wanted to light the candles for a procession; she had no matches; however, seeing the little lamp which was burning in front of the relics, she

approached it. Alas, it was half out; there remained only a feeble glimmer on its blackened wick. She succeeded in lighting her candle from it, and with this candle, she lighted those of the whole community. It was, therefore, the half-extinguished little lamp which has produced all these beautiful flames which, in their turn, could produce an infinity of others and even light the whole universe. Nevertheless, it would always be the little lamp which would be first cause of all this light. How could the beautiful flames boast of having produced this fire, when they themselves were lighted with such a small spark?[4]

Thérèse's life reflected these paradoxical themes. While experiencing the great physical, emotional, and spiritual suffering associated with late-stage tuberculosis, Thérèse lifted up everyone around her. She projected a strength of character that her sisters described as both generous and heroic. At the same time, Thérèse fully acknowledged her fears, and even what she saw as her cowardice:

> I've been told so much that I have courage, and this is so far from the truth, that I have said to myself: Well, then, you mustn't make a liar out of everybody! And so I set myself, with the help of grace, to the acquisition of courage. I've acted just like a warrior who, hearing himself always being praised for his bravery, and knowing that he's nothing but a coward, ends up by being ashamed of the compliments and wants to be deserving of them.[5]

Just as she sought to spare others pain, Thérèse practiced a sustained form of understated strength that represented a monumental expression of the "little way." As her sister Pauline noted, even as Thérèse was contemplating her own death, "She was thinking of us."[6]

Thinking of others can represent a striking expression of courage and faith at the end of life. In his best-selling book *Being Mortal: Medicine and What Matters in the End*, the surgeon Atul Gawande has described courage as the endurance of the soul.[7] Gawande has noted that this form of power can be vital both to the person and to those around them. The sociologist Allan Kellehear has similarly observed that showing "courage in the face of death" engages "the preservation and protection of those things and people one cherishes—foundational personal values, friends, family, country—and the dignity, social bonds, cherished reciprocity, and self-identity that are embedded in these crucial relationships."[8] The palliative care physician Harvey Max Chochinov has also characterized expressions of resilience and the fighting spirit as examples of a dignity conserving perspective, and he has described spiritual comfort as a dignity conserving practice.[9]

While working in Acute Palliative Care, I am privileged to be present while people tell stories of courage and faith. One day I met a remarkable mother and daughter. The mother lay in bed, actively dying, while I spoke quietly with the daughter at her bedside. The woman told me that, while her mother was now nonresponsive, a few days prior they had an important conversation that affirmed their family legacy:

"I'm Okay With This": My Mother's Daughter

In our lives, when something hard would come up,
My mother would always say, "I'm okay with this."
That was her thing.
My mother has a strong faith,
And she is at peace.

Three days ago she called me over to her and said,
"Mamma's got to talk to you now.
Mamma's going away.
I'm okay with this.
And now, I need to know
That you're okay with this, too.
I need you to tell me this."

And I did.
I am my mother's daughter.

The woman then shared that, saying these words aloud was one of the most difficult things that she ever had to do in her life. Because she found the strength to affirm her "okay-ness" with the situation, her mother was able to let go with peace and grace. Such an exchange not only required enormous courage, but it created an even deeper sense of continuity between how the women lived their lives, and how they faced the end of life together. Through their mutual affirmations of courage and continuity, the younger woman indeed showed herself to be her mother's daughter.

In a reversal yet mirroring of this story, one mother proudly observed of her dying daughter:

She Made Me Strong, As Well

My daughter cares for people a great deal.
She was always smiling,
Even when things were horrible—
You'd never know it.
She wanted us to have a positive attitude.

Her faith is so strong.
Through all of this, she's had the strength.
And, she's made me strong, as well.

Even as she lay actively dying, the slight young woman strengthened everyone around her. These themes also arose the day I visited with a very young man who suffered from an aggressive glioblastoma. As he lay in his hospital bed, his mother recounted the principal events of her son's brief life. She proudly concluded:

My son confronted this illness like nobody else.
Everyone who knows him says the same thing.
He never gave up.
He has a lot of patience,
And he's a good spirit,
And very brave.
My son's life is all about courage and faith.
He is a warrior.

While the young man had great difficulty speaking and he could no longer see out of one eye, as he heard the story he called over and affirmed: "It's perfect. Go ahead. Absolutely share this." Another brave young woman combined the themes of the warrior and the cross as she addressed her own mortality. While she suffered from an extremely aggressive sarcoma of the jaw, this young woman still managed to retain her beautiful smile. Her strong sense of faith became evident in the interwoven themes of her artwork, which centered on her love for God and her mother:

Made of Gold: The Ribbon and the Cross

My images are the ribbon—the symbol for cancer—and the cross.
The ribbon is a sign of me surviving,
Being strong and fighting,
And of me overcoming.
This is a part of who I am.

For me, the cross is my getaway.
I turn to church, and to the Bible.
Going to church is one of my favorite things.
The cross symbolizes my life.
And, it gives me the strength to impact other people's lives.

My mom strengthens me.
She gives me comfort and tells me I'm never alone,
That God is with me.
Her smile lights up the room,
And it makes me feel like gold.

As we worked together, the young woman's mother sat at the foot of the hospital bed. After I read the words aloud, the mother thanked me and responded:

My daughter is a fighter.
She's a go-getter, very independent and strong.
She always befriended other people.
And, her love of God has intensified even more.

God Had My Back: Finding Courage Through Divine Connection

While some people describe the ways in which they draw strength from their families, others will recount their perception of a divine presence that fortified them in times of hardship. One woman told me how she felt such a presence as she handled a dangerous situation at work. As she said:

God took me to that job.
I know that's where God wanted me to be.
God opened doors with the supervisors to get me hired.
There was a bad situation there,
And I cleaned it up.
The managers said they'd back me up,
And they stood by me.
God gave me the strength to stand up and not back down.

I stood strong because, I knew God held my hand,
And He had my back.

Even since I was a child,
I was not afraid.
I knew God had my back.

One man literally described the sense of courage he felt in knowing that God had his back. This very quiet man was a First Responder. In fact, he was so quiet that you would never know how heroic he was. It was only in my drawing him out that his extraordinary bravery came to light. As we visited, he told a story of courage and faith while serving others:

Making An Impact: His Hand on My Back

I'm retired now,
But I was a police officer.
I did many things.
I worked on the Marine Unit, with boats and helicopters.
I did search and rescue work.
I always had the feeling that I would be a police officer.
I was always very observant, and I always wanted to help people.
I always wanted to be making an impact,
Especially with saving a life.
It's why I wanted to be out on the marine vessels.

Over my career, I've saved over a hundred lives.
It feels great to know you made a difference,

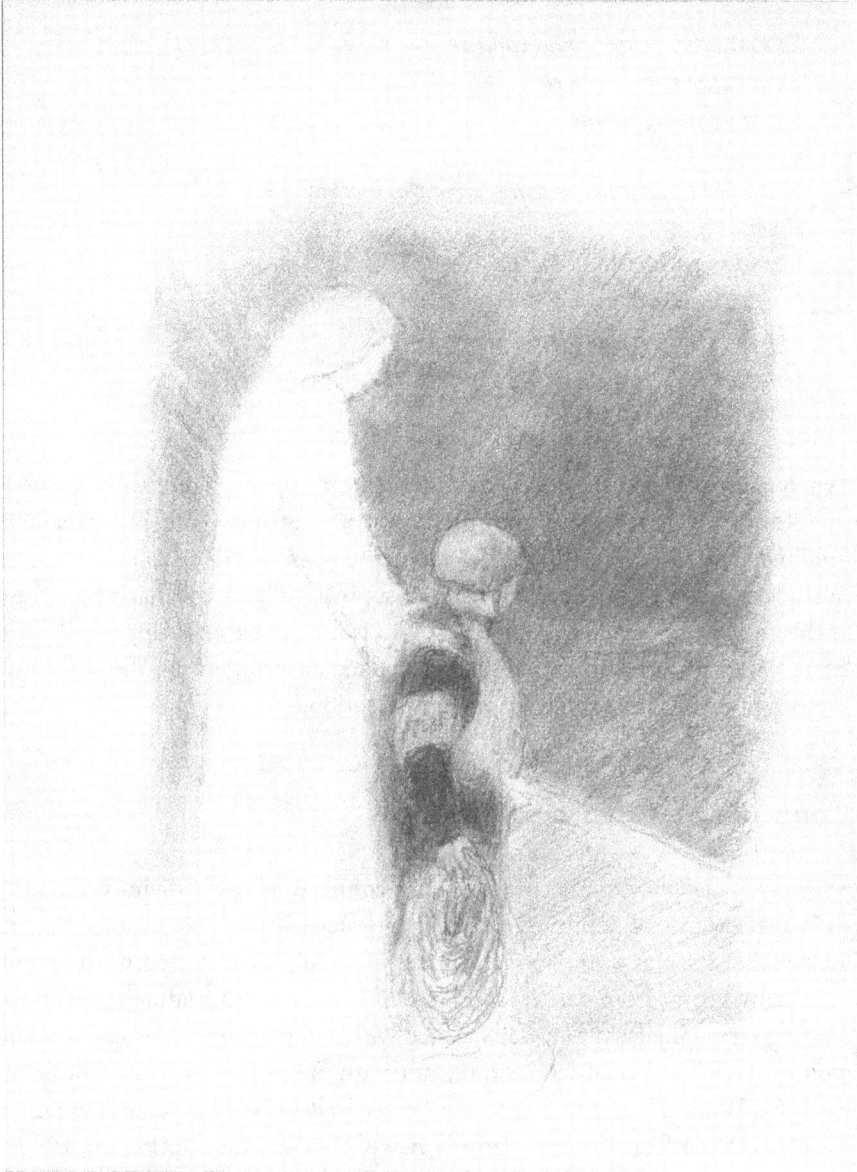

Figure 24: Lyn Smallwood, *His Hand on My Back*, 2021, graphite on white Strathmore drawing paper

So that other people could continue their life,
Despite the risks involved.
It's an amazing feeling.

Did I feel a spiritual presence doing this work?
Absolutely.
I would just reach out and say,
"God, please give me the strength to get through this.
I know You have Your hand on my back."
On some occasions, I can tell you,
I really did feel His hand.

Lyn Smallwood's illustration, *His Hand on My Back* (Figure 24), shows a middle-aged policeman standing in uniform, wearing a life preserver and holding a coiled rope. Behind him stands the open, luminous silhouette of a much larger figure whose radiant hands rest powerfully on the man's back. Just as this presence is subtle and etheric, so too is it palpable and supportive. This unseen force gave the man strength as he looked outward toward the water and prepared to enter yet another dangerous situation.

Connections with Sacred Presences

Sometimes people express such personal connections with divinity through their perceptions of subtle presences. For others, formal expressions of religious belief serve as foundational sources of strength and support. These can take many forms, from participating in religious rituals to reading scripture or viewing sacred imagery. One day I visited with a middle-aged Mexican woman who expressed a special connection, not with Saint Thérèse, but with Saint Faustina. While Thérèse of Lisieux has been a well-known figure for more than a century, Saint Faustina is a relatively new Catholic saint. During the 1930s, Faustina Kowalska was a humble young Polish nun who received revelations concerning divine mercy and the Misericordia (which is the Latin term for mercy, as associated with the heart). Sister Faustina recorded these insights in her notebooks, which were later published. Faustina was canonized by Pope John Paul II in 2000.

Since the woman in the hospital primarily spoke Spanish, her sister served as a translator, and she also contributed to the narrative. The woman at the end of life told me that she and her family belonged to a charismatic Catholic church, and that they performed special devotions to Saint Faustina.[10] As the women spoke admiringly of the saint, I recorded their vision of

Saint Faustina: The Mercy of the Broken Heart

There's something special for me in the connection with Saint Faustina.
The connection is through the Misericordia—
The broken heart—
Which took the form of a brooch of the heart
That Christ gave her in devotion.
An image was later painted of her vision.
Saint Faustina is a nun of faith,
And this is what takes us in.

We found our church, and then she got sick.
Since knowing of this sickness,
We've been praying the rosary for one year.
Every time we pray, she is lifted up,
And He takes away the pain.
Every day, Jesus has a connection with her.
She always has God by her hand.

When I knew I was sick, I was so prepared in my faith.
It brings the family to church.
Faith brings the family together,
And it is part of Jesus.
There's a special rosary for the Misericordia,
And, there's always forgiveness.

Such narratives raise compelling questions regarding the role that saints such as Faustina or Thérèse can play in what the sociologist and novelist Andrew Greeley has called "the Catholic imagination." For Greeley, the term refers broadly to an individual's perception of living in an enchanted world, where creation is seen as a mark of sacred presence. As Greeley notes, such perceptions can inspire "a sense that the objects, events, and persons of daily life are revelations of grace."[11] In this case, the words and images of Saint Faustina helped the women to conceptualize the humanity of divinity, just as they brought the heaven world closer to home during a period of pronounced pain and hardship. For this family, the Misericordia of Saint Faustina provided a sacred image of a broken heart that strengthened the collective power of all of their hearts.

To You, I Leave My Heart: The Strength of the Heart at the End of Life

Thérèse's first practical experience of attending a person at the end of life was also deeply informed by the imagery of the heart. In December of 1891, while still a teenager, Thérèse assisted at the death of an elderly nun named Mother Geneviève. This was Thérèse's first experience with an actual death, and it represented an act of courage and care. As Thérèse recalled, "the spectacle was ravishing" and "the memory which Mother Geneviève left in my heart is a sacred memory." After standing at the foot of the bed for two hours, Thérèse experienced "an inexpressible joy and fervor," and she had the paradoxical mystical insight that a death on earth is also a "birth in heaven," an event that marked the ongoing life of the soul. After Mother Geneviève's passing, Thérèse recalled a dream that featured a sacred memory of the heart. As she wrote: "I dreamed [Mother Geneviève] was making her last will and testament, giving each of the Sisters something which she possessed. When my turn finally came, I thought I would get nothing as there was really nothing left to give; however, she said: 'To you, I leave my *heart.*' She repeated this three times with great emphasis."[12] Thérèse was thus gifted with a mystical dream of the heart. Resonating with this imagery, a statue of the Blessed Virgin Mary with an exposed heart stood in the convent garden at the Carmel of Lisieux (Figure 25). This devotional image shows the Immaculate Heart of Mary as an emblem of her sorrows, her joys, and her compassionate presence. In such imagery, the heart appears as a sign of mystical corporeality that unites human beings and sacred presences.

In end-of-life narratives, images of courage and enduring life are often associated with the strength of the heart. On various levels, this is fitting. Just as the heart appears as a symbol of faith and fortitude, the term "courage" stems from the Latin root *cor*, which literally denotes the heart. One day I met a man who was fully oriented yet extremely close to death. His metastatic prostate cancer had spread to his bones, and his hip was hurting so badly that tears of pain came to his eyes every time he shifted his position in bed. Even as the team worked to control his refractory symptoms, the man shared an extremely beautiful narrative of

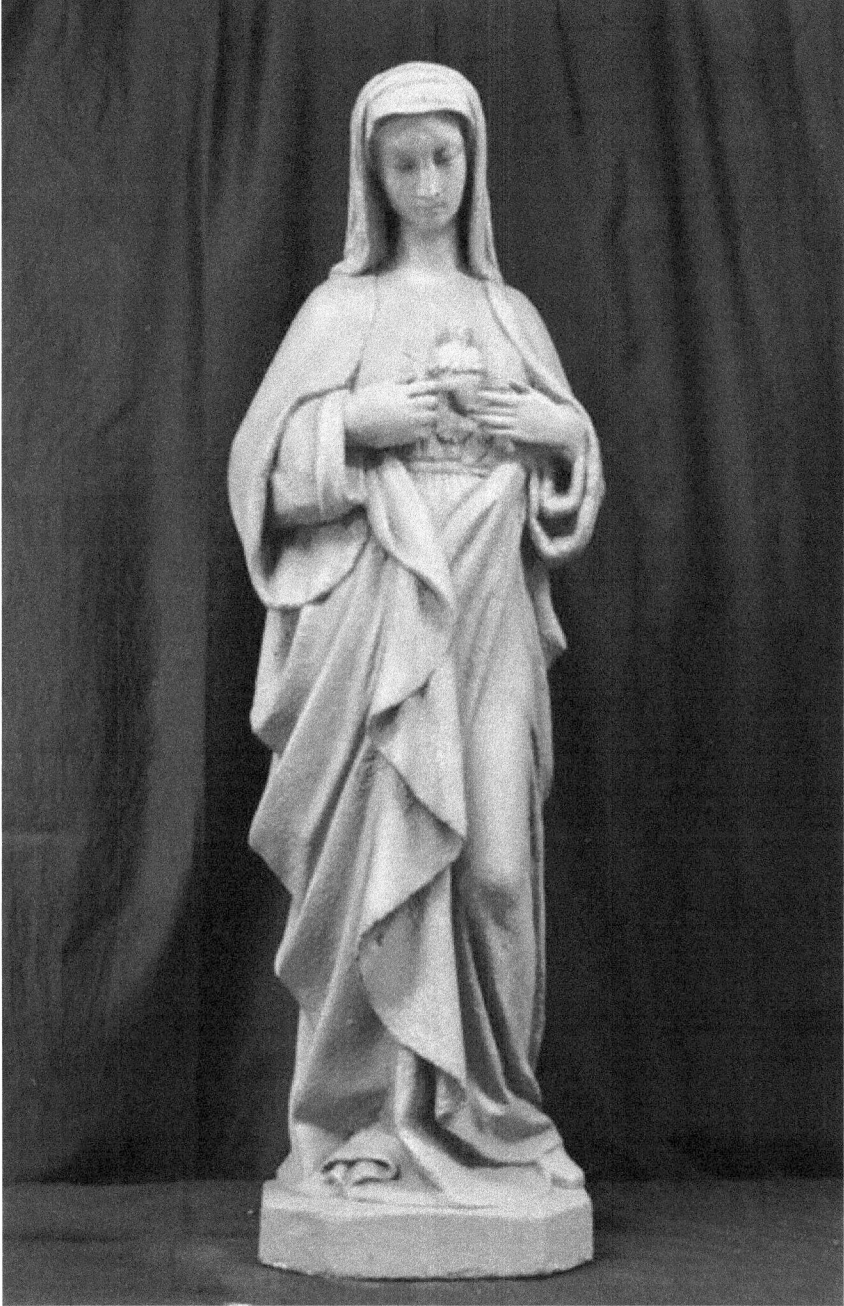

Figure 25: Statue of the Virgin of the Garden, Convent at the Carmel of Lisieux.
© Archives du Carmel de Lisieux, http://www.archives-carmel-lisieux.fr/

The Beating Heart

My image is of my family and friends.
My family has been there for me since I was born.
But first in my family is God.
He's always been there for me.
I am so blessed.
I see how good He has been to me.

I see Him as a spirit.
If you put a picture on it,
It would look like a heart,
Like a beating human heart,
With the aorta pumping.
That's the lifeline that keeps you going.

God comes in so many forms.
When a person goes into cardiac arrest,
The heart stops beating.
And when babies are born,
The first thing they do is to get the heart started beating.
If the heart doesn't beat,
We've lost a life.

I share these images with my family.
We all have the same beating heart.

Ultimately, the man passed away a few days after our visit. But on that day, while he faced the end of his life, he was able to feel the palpable presence of God each time his own heart contracted.

From One Heart to Another: The Doublings that Unite Worlds

I was there the day the news finally arrived. Unfortunately, the prognosis was grim. The young man was told that his melanoma had metastasized and that he was no longer eligible to receive treatment. His parents, who themselves were still quite young, were gathered at his bedside. They openly acknowledged the difficulty they faced in trying to process this news. These circumstances made

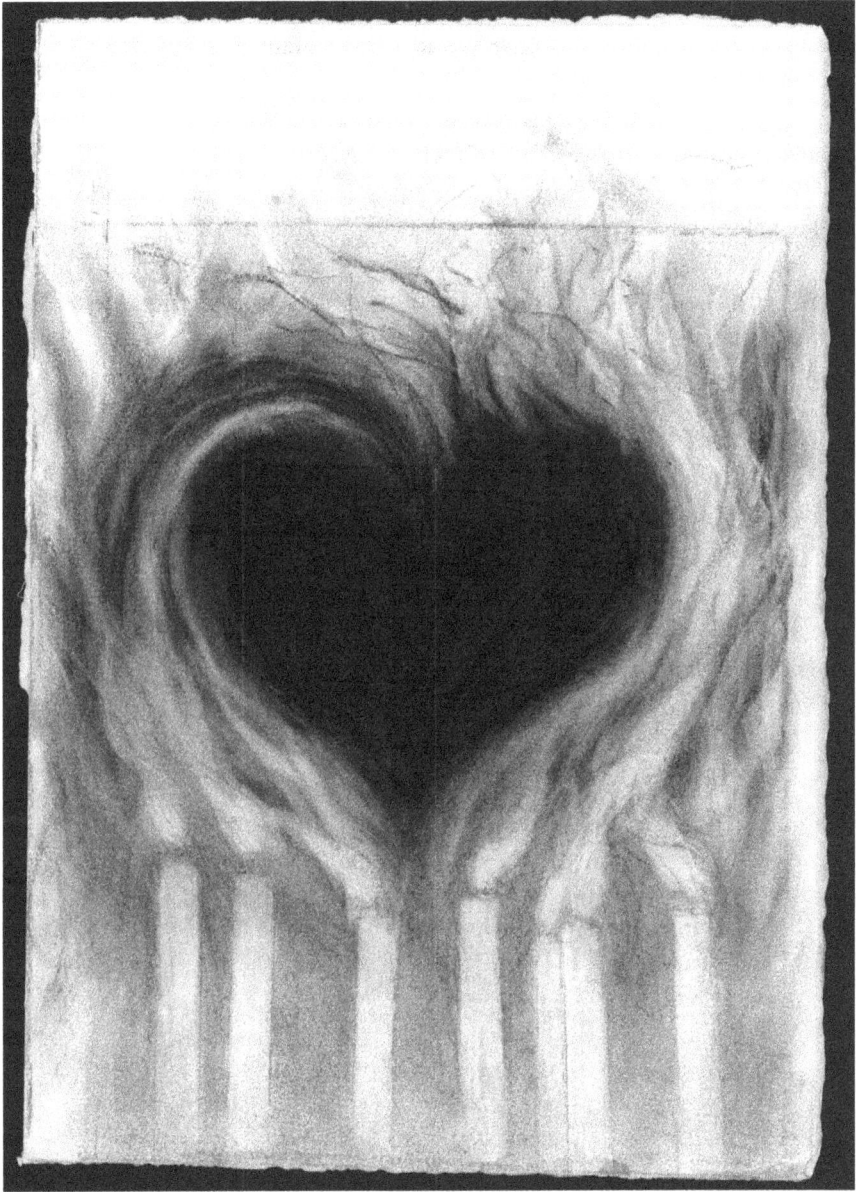

Figure 26: Lyn Smallwood, *From One Heart to Another*, 2012, charcoal on white Canson paper

for a very intense and moving visit, and I am so grateful to have been present on that day of all days.

As we visited, the young man drew a picture of a heart, which he then shaded in various tones of red, and which he surrounded with bright yellow rays of light. After contemplating the image, the young man sketched seven candles along the bottom edge of the drawing. Sitting atop a grassy green path, the candles resembled square red bricks topped with golden flames. While he worked on the drawing, the young man described his understanding of how power radiates

From One Heart to Another

I draw a big heart
Because that's where your soul is
And it radiates from that point.
It radiates to all the good in my life,
To family and friends.
The light is not just radiating out.
It's also radiating in.
It's a reflection,
A reflection of God.

You see that light
From one heart to another.
I see this in the faith in my life,
In my Christianity,
In my belief.
It's in the candles,
And in the flames.

In my mind,
I'm seeing that there are seven red candles
For seven days of the week.
I put up a seven day fight,
And the fight never ends.

The young man was clearly working hard to remain strong for his family, yet everyone was close to tears as both the news and the imagery were so close to all of their hearts. In these difficult circumstances, the young man's artwork appears as both a statement of faith and an affirmation of love. Through his symbolic imagery, life itself appears as a kind of devotional offering, a vision that holds all things within a shared light. Hearing his son's words, the father poignantly responded that people say that the eyes are the windows of the soul, but that his son may be right, the heart is the window of the Lord.

Lyn Smallwood's charcoal drawing, *From One Heart to Another* (Figure 26), depicts the young man's expressive themes of courage, faith, flames, and spirit. Seven tall candles appear along the bottom edge of the drawing. Each of the lit tapers is topped by a flame with dark smoke that curls upward and inward to form the shape of a heart. Perched above the candles, the velvety black image of the heart is literally constructed of charcoal, an artistic medium that is produced from burnt matter. Dark and solid yet swirling and diaphanous, the image of the heart rising from the flames appears to be powerful even as it is evanescent. Through these images, the artwork bridges the distance from one heart to another as it presents a reciprocal exchange of rising and falling light.

Notes

1. Orsi, *History and Presence*, 164, 214. In this volume, Orsi presents extended discussions of the various conceptions of sacred presence that emerged within the social and cultural histories of twentieth-century Catholicism, which placed considerable emphasis on the relations between the dead and the living.

2. David Morgan, *The Lure of Images: A History of Religion and Visual Media in America* (New York: Routledge, 2007), 251, 255.

3. Quoted in *St. Thérèse of Lisieux*, 142.

4. Quoted in *St. Thérèse of Lisieux*, 99.

5. Quoted in *St. Thérèse of Lisieux*, 48.

6. Quoted in *St. Thérèse of Lisieux*, 58.

7. Atul Gawande, *Being Mortal: Medicine and What Matters in the End* (New York: Picador, 2017), 231.

8. Allan Kellehear, *The Inner Life of the Dying Person* (New York: Columbia University Press, 2014), 70–71.

9. Harvey Max Chochinov, *Dignity Therapy: Final Words for Final Days* (New York: Oxford University Press, 2012), 9. Chochinov advocates dignity therapy as an "end of life planning tool" associated with promoting the will to live among terminally ill people.

10. This story exemplifies the ways in which particular images of saints can provide powerful sources of strength and faith when facing extreme hardships. Yet Orsi notes that a degree of caution should be exercised when an afflicted person with real human needs and desires becomes identified with the sufferings of a particular saint or holy figure. As he has observed, through strategies of appropriation and inversion, the saint can become an ambivalent sign that affirms the suffering person's own presence. Just as suffering saints can make suffering human beings more visible to themselves and to others, identification with a particular saint can also serve as a form of appropriation in which the holy person becomes a sign of the suffering person's own presence. Such practices can be used for the enforcement, or for the potential subversion, of established social norms and identities. Thus Orsi underscores the need to be attentive to the complex issues of power and agency that can arise when vulnerable populations are cast into particular social roles. See Orsi, *Between Heaven and Earth*, 1–4, 46.

11. Andrew Greeley, *The Catholic Imagination* (Berkeley: University of California Press, 2000), 1, 18. Just as Greeley acknowledges that not all Catholics are deeply affected by this conception of the Catholic imagination, he also recognizes that people other than Catholics see creation as sacred.
12. Quoted in *Story of a Soul*, 170–71.

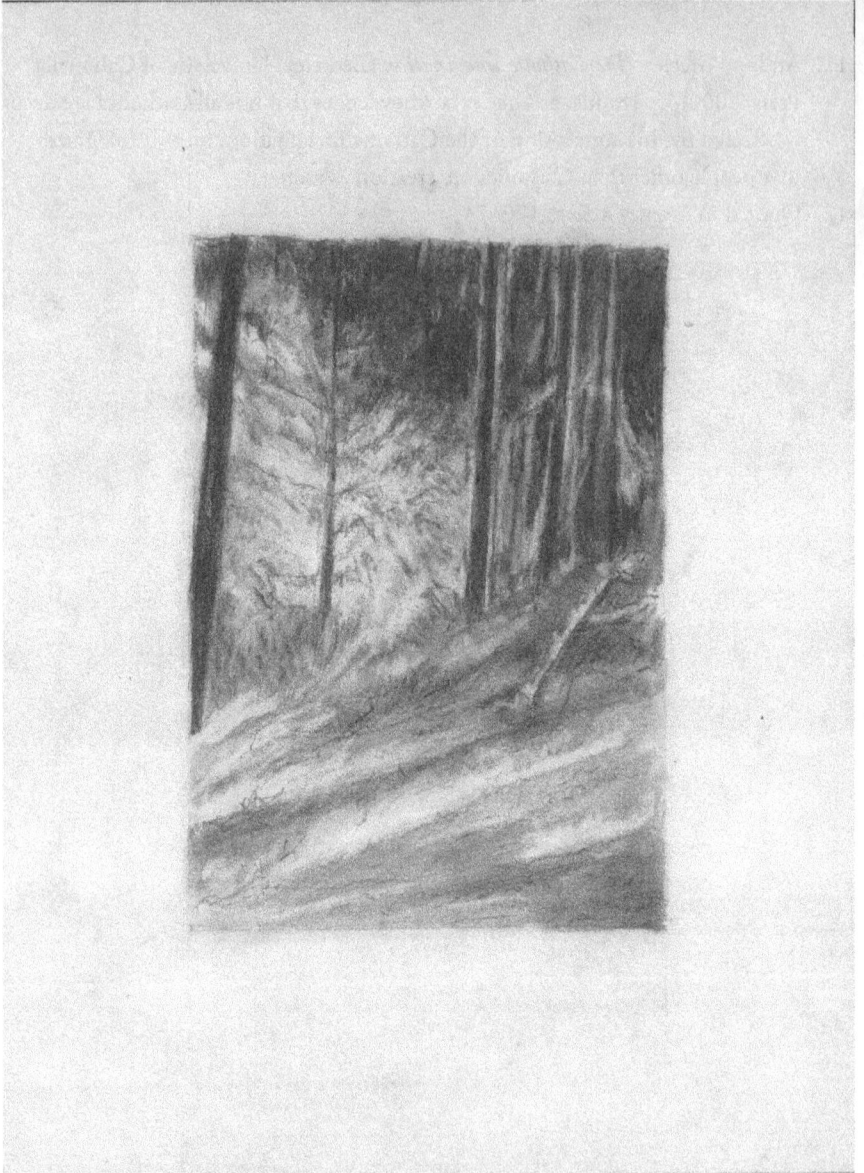

Figure 27: Lyn Smallwood, *Beneath the Trees*, 2020, graphite on white Strathmore drawing paper

Chapter Seven

Kissing the Void: Vision and Blindness as the Two Sides of the Veil

Beneath the Trees: Stories of Shadows, and of Lights

One day I met an older woman who sat all alone in her hospital room. While the medical team found her to be somewhat critical and demanding—particularly in her desire for strict adherence to the details of a daily routine—I found the woman to be extremely candid and forthright. Early in the visit, she told me matter-of-factly that she "had a tragic life." She also expressed her appreciation for the care and kindness she received from the clinical team. As we spoke together, various elements of her life story emerged. Ultimately, we produced two narratives. The tone of the first story is extremely somber, as the woman's imagery transitions from light to darkness, from life to death:

Beneath the Trees

My sister died of exactly the same type of cancer that I'm dying of,
So I have a real picture of what this is,
And what is coming.

Our family is from Switzerland.
When my sister was at the hospital in Switzerland,
An art therapist would come twice a week to work with her.
My sister was a gifted and prolific artist
And you could see the progression of the imagery.

In the beginning, my sister's pictures were very colorful,
With lush trees and lots of green leaves.
At the end, the pictures were more abstract.
There was a lot of black.

There were leaves falling everywhere,
And there was a fire with a lot of orange
Burning beneath the trees.

Lyn Smallwood's intricate pencil landscape, *Beneath the Trees* (Figure 27), reflects key aspects of this difficult story. This darkly elegiac artwork evokes a harrowing sense of loss. The scene depicts a forest in a state of destruction, with leaves falling and fires burning beneath the trees. With its tenor of desolation, the artwork presents an image of a dying world rather than a living one. Yet as our visit unfolded, the woman's sense of sorrow became modified by a new insight. As she reflected further on the members of her family, the woman began to discern a subtle presence in her life. These themes emerged in her subsequent narrative:

She Will Be There

When you asked about my imagery,
The picture that immediately came to mind is that,
I have a little gold ring with four diamonds at the top.

I had dated a guy for many years, and we broke up.
It was very sad.
Afterwards, I wrote to my cousin in Switzerland.
This is my godmother's daughter.
One year she sent me a Christmas card,
And in the envelope there was an itty bitty piece of bubble wrap,
With this ring inside.

It belonged to my godmother.
When she died, her older son sold all her jewelry.
But this wedding band was on her hand.
My cousin said, "You should have this, if anybody.
You were very close to my mother.
She would want you to have it."

It was one of the nicest, kindest things
Anyone ever did for me,
To give me that ring.

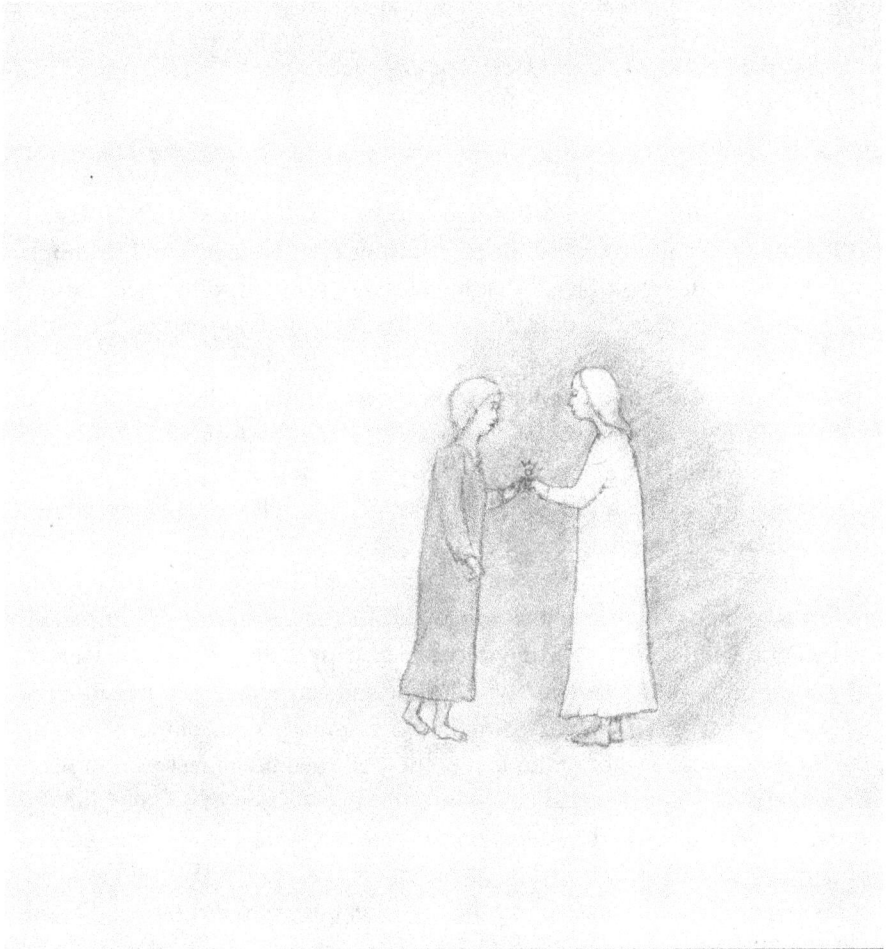

Figure 28: Lyn Smallwood, *She Will Be There*, 2020, graphite on white Strathmore drawing paper

This ring has always been special to me.
But now, telling this story makes me think that,
When I cross over,
She will be there.

While *Beneath the Trees* is detailed and naturalistic, *She Will Be There* (Figure 28) is minimal and schematic. In this drawing, two women stand in profile facing one another. Soft pencil shading creates a gentle haloing effect around their etheric silhouettes. A gold ring with four diamonds appears at the center of the image; this object serves as both a material and a symbolic point of connection between the two women and the worlds they inhabit. During our visit, the ring provided a tangible presence for the dying woman to hold onto as she envisioned a reunion with her beloved godmother. This insight greatly comforted the woman and brought her perspective full circle, like the golden ring that forms the centerpiece of this story.

When taken together, the woman's narratives follow a trajectory from life to death to life again, just as they forge a connection between multiple states of being. Beginning with her raw account of pain and suffering, the woman was able to transition to a sense of gratitude and accompaniment because she consciously recognized the magnitude of a seemingly small thing. Recalling the love of someone who was no longer there allowed her to feel a warm sense of connection, which enabled her to imagine a new vision of ongoing life. By engaging these themes, the stories can be seen as complementary expressions of darkness and light, fear and faith, blindness and vision. These subjects are central not only to the culture of palliative care, but to the writings of Thérèse of Lisieux.

Going Behind the Curtain: Subtle Knowledge, Blindness, and Vision

From an early point in her life, veiled worlds appeared as sheltered spaces where Thérèse experienced a sense of spiritual connection. As a child, Thérèse knew the charm of being in the world, yet she also imagined being a hermit and a blind person. These games allowed her to practice living in multiple worlds at once. At the age of eight, Thérèse and her cousin, Marie Guérin, played games of Thérèse's invention in which

Marie and Thérèse became two *hermits*, having nothing but a poor hut, a little garden where they grew corn and other vegetables. Their life was spent in continual contemplation; in other words, one *hermit* replaced the other at prayer while she was occupied in the active life. Everything was done with such mutual understanding, silence, and so religiously that it was just perfect. When Aunt came to fetch us to go for our walks, we continued the game even on the street.

Cousin Marie and I were always of the same opinion and our tastes were so much the same that once our *union of wills* passed all bounds. Returning one evening from the Abbey, I said to Marie: "Lead me, I'm going to close my eyes." "I want to close mine, too," she replied. No sooner said than done; without *arguing*, each did her *will*. We were on a sidewalk and there was nothing to fear from vehicles; having savored the delights of walking without seeing, the two little scamps fell *together* on some cases placed at the door of a store, or rather they tipped them over. The merchant came out in a rage to lift up his merchandise, while the two blind ones lifted themselves up alone and walked off *at great strides, eyes wide open*.[1]

Like Thérèse, Marie would later become a Carmelite nun. In their childhood games, Thérèse and Marie practiced alternate ways of being in the world, of relying on senses other than sight while going behind the veil of their closed eyelids. In youthful moments of solitude, Thérèse also went behind a bed curtain where she envisioned an alternate reality and engaged in silent prayer. In *Story of a Soul* Thérèse recalled how, in childhood, she was taught to make vocal prayers but not interior ones. When one of her teachers asked Thérèse how she spent her free afternoons at home, the little girl responded:

I told her I went behind my bed in an empty space which was there, and that it was easy to close myself in with my bed curtain and that "*I thought*." "But what do you think about?" she asked. "I think about God, about life, about ETERNITY ... I *think*!" The good religious laughed heartily at me, and later on she loved reminding me of the time when I *thought*, asking me if *I was still thinking*. I understand now that I was making mental prayer without knowing it and that God was already instructing me in secret.[2]

While recounting this experience, Thérèse explained how she instinctively entered a world within a world as she sat in the liminal space between the wall and the bed curtain. In this enclosed area, Thérèse found a passageway for divine communication. Whether her childhood activities unfolded within the shelter of a pretend hermitage, or beneath her own closed eyes, or under the veil of her bed curtain, Thérèse repeatedly explored passing through boundaries to explore states of vision and blindness.

Later in life, as a Discalced Carmelite nun Thérèse not only wore the veil that distinguished the habit of her order, but she drew on the imagery of curtains and veils, of knowing and not knowing, as she described her connection with divine presence. While working in the convent refectory, Thérèse recalled her sense of entering such a sacred world:

> It was as though a veil had been cast over all the things of this earth for me … I was entirely hidden under the Blessed Virgin's veil. At this time, I was placed in charge of the refectory, and I recall doing things as though not doing them; it was as if someone had lent me a body. I remained that way for one whole week.[3]

As both a human being and a future saint, Thérèse's life was filled with the imagery of lights and shadows, vision and blindness. Just as these ambivalent themes are the hallmark of a mystical tradition,[4] they became pronounced as Thérèse faced the end of her life. As she imagined her own death, she speculated apprehensively on the "tearing of the veil" that marks the separation of the body and the soul. When speaking with her sister Pauline two months before her passing, Thérèse recounted a particular verse in Saint John of the Cross's *The Living Flame of Love*: "Tear through the veil of this sweet encounter!" Thérèse then shared the meanings that these words held for her: "I've always applied these words to the death of love that I desire. Love will not wear out the veil of my life; it will tear suddenly."[5] Thérèse thus characterized her human life as a veil that covered her soul, a fabric that would rip abruptly at life's culmination.

Even as she had such visionary knowledge, Thérèse still suffered greatly. At the end of her life, she experienced air hunger and the agony of suffocation associated with advanced tuberculosis. She admitted that she didn't know how to die, and she prayed that she could die immediately because she was experiencing unbearable physical suffering. When confronting the harsh reality of her own death, Thérèse openly admitted, "I am afraid I have feared death. I am not afraid of what happens after death; that is certain! I don't regret giving up my life; but I ask myself: What is this mysterious separation of the soul from the body? It is the first time that I have experienced this, but I abandoned myself immediately to God … It is into God's arms that I'm falling!"[6]

Related themes arise in contemporary end of life imagery. Sometimes people suffer so greatly that they are blindsided by their experiences, unable to see life clearly or to cope with what is unfolding all around them. I will share three such stories of the shadows, in which people are overwhelmed by trauma.

Blindsided: Being Beside Oneself

One day I entered a room where a man was actively dying. While this was certainly not an unusual occurrence on the Acute Palliative Care Inpatient Unit, what *was* unusual was how the man's family and friends were responding—with an intense mixture of love, denial, and desperation. During the hour and a half that I spent in that room, the man went from being minimally responsive, with mild but visible symptoms of agitation and delirium, to entering into a state of actively dying as his breathing became labored and the characteristic "death rattle" emanated from his throat. Instead of acknowledging that the man was at the end of his life, the family frantically started making phone calls and texting people, so that more and more people entered the room. As people kept pouring in, the man's wife repeatedly went up to his bedside and tried to rouse him and have him interact with the new arrivals. The visitors smiled nervously and they kept asking the man if he wanted anything to eat or drink, or if he wanted to sit up, etc. Almost everyone struggled to treat the man as if he were still conscious, even going so far as to make jokes with him and carry on life as usual. These actions only increased the man's agitation and made everyone feel more strained, unsettled, and frightened.

On that afternoon, I sat at the juncture of life and death as I watched a conflicting drama unfold. The man was clearly ready to die and what he needed was peace and quiet, and his family's acceptance of the situation. Yet his well-meaning family responded in just the opposite way, as they futilely attempted to pull him back into the world and back into their lives. When their narrative was complete I informed the medical team of the situation, noting that the man was clearly ready to die and that his family and friends were unable to let him go. The charge nurse told me that the physician would speak to them and let them know that the man needed to rest. This would serve as a kind of compromise position that would buy some time, while giving the family an opportunity to recognize for themselves what was occurring. In other words, this gentle medical intervention could create a space between worlds.

Almost remarkably, I have only encountered such extremely difficult situations a handful of times. I will share a few more examples, because the stories demonstrate how people can become so overwhelmed that their thoughts and actions become distorted and words and reason fail them. The next story expresses these sentiments viscerally in a narrative entitled *You Make Me Sick!*

A middle-aged woman lay at the end of her life, tossing in bed in a state of pronounced delirium while the team worked hard at getting her symptoms under control. I knocked softly on the door and introduced myself as an Artist In Residence. No sooner had these words left my mouth when the patient's mother, who was sitting in the chair nearest the door, sprang out of her seat and physically lunged at me. In a state of uncontrolled rage, she snarled and said, "You make me sick! Leave this room immediately!" It took me a moment to process what was happening, as nothing like this had ever occurred before, and there was no apparent reason for such a violent response. I quietly left the room and reported the incident to the attending nurse and the social worker, who were equally puzzled. The social worker went into the room to try to make sense of what had just happened. Speaking with the woman, he was able to discern that she had mistakenly thought I was a visual artist who was there to make drawings of her dying daughter, which I would sell for profit on the Internet. While the social worker clarified the role of the Artist In Residence service in general, the woman remained in a state of rage, unable to hear anything further.

On another day, I met a middle-aged woman who was a practicing physician in China. She had brought her young son to M.D. Anderson to receive treatment that could not be obtained elsewhere. Sadly, the treatments for his extremely aggressive intestinal cancer proved to be ineffective, and the young man was actively dying. Because the family was Mandarin-speaking only, I collaborated with the hospital interpreter, who introduced me as an Artist In Residence and, at my request, asked the woman to tell me something wonderful about her son. The woman angrily questioned who I was and why I was there at all. She insisted that neither she nor her son believed in God or the afterlife, and she asked me to leave, which I did. It was apparent that the woman felt that the hospital had failed her, and she was nearly hysterical with grief and rage. Much like the woman who had exclaimed: "You make me sick!," this mother was perilously close to being out of control, and she represented a danger both to herself and to those around her. Once again, I left the room and reported the incident to the patient's nurse and to the counselor, the latter of whom agreed with my assessment, and who told me that the woman struggled to cope by demanding further, futile medical treatments, which were not to be forthcoming.

These narratives all tell stories of vision and blindness. Each expresses a state of consciousness that surpasses the boundaries of reason and language, as people are so overwhelmed by a situation that they are engulfed in grief and rage, sadness and fear. Such individuals are literally beside themselves as they confront the unknown. While the stories relate depths of pain that can never be fully expressed, they also provide insight into extreme states of human experience. Paradoxically, such narratives are the opposite *and* the complement of the stories of light, faith, and joy that appear elsewhere in this book. Despite their notable differences, both types of narratives represent expressions of ecstasy. According to *Webster's Seventh New Collegiate Dictionary*, ecstasy literally denotes a condition of standing outside of oneself. The term descends from the Greek, *ekstasis*, which combines the prefix *ex* (or "out") with the root *histanai*, which signifies "to cause to stand." The definitions of the term encompass a broad emotional spectrum as a person experiences overwhelming emotions that lead to "a state of being beyond reason and self-control." Such responses can range from "rapturous delight," transport, and exaltation to the "overmastering emotions" of rage and fear.[7]

End-of-life narratives reflect this broad emotional spectrum. While doing this work, I have frequently witnessed the ways in which transcendence can connect the deepest suffering with the highest joy. Both states are boundless, as the ground drops out from under our feet and the sky opens over our heads. Both states can inspire an extreme sense of humility at the privilege of being present. As both terror and joy dismantle the familiar boundaries between worlds, these experiences can literally leave us floored. Both states can create radical openings, just as they appear as opposites that are not always opposite. In their sheer magnitude, the experiences allow us to be present among something greater than ourselves. Such extreme states of abjection and elation, suffering and joy, require us to acknowledge the part of our humanity that lies beyond the boundaries of language, the part that exceeds what can ever be fully known by or about another human being.

The Table of Sorrow and the Night of Nothingness: Thérèse's Trial of Faith

In her accounts of praying behind the bed curtain and being "hidden under the Blessed Virgin's veil," Thérèse described a state of being enclosed within a permeable membrane that fostered a sense of protection and union with divine presence. In these narratives, the veil appears as a kind of connective tissue that provides access to the numinous. Yet just as Thérèse cherished these associations, she also had a veiled mystical experience in which a boundary was placed between herself and the heavenly world, a barrier that thrust her deeply into the shadows of despair. Before the onset of this great trial, Thérèse recalled how her end-of-life experience began with a sense of joy that preceded pronounced bitterness. In the night between Holy Thursday and Good Friday of 1896, when Thérèse laid her head down on the pillow to go to sleep, she "felt something like a bubbling stream mounting to my lips." In the darkness she did not know what the substance was, but in the morning light her suspicions were confirmed and she realized that "it was blood I had coughed up."[8] This was her first hemoptysis, an airway bleeding that marked the initial sign of the tuberculosis that would claim Thérèse's life a year and a half later.

Her first response was rejoicing at the thought that she would soon be going to heaven. As she recalled, "At this time I was enjoying such a living faith, such a clear *faith*, that the thought of heaven made up all my happiness, and I was unable to believe that there really were impious people who had no faith." Shortly thereafter, Thérèse experienced a trial of faith that would last until her death. In *Story of a Soul*, she famously recalled being led to a place of despair where she encountered souls who were devoid of all faith and who saw death only as "the night of nothingness." Thérèse described this darkly mystical image:

> During those very joyful days of the Easter season, Jesus made me feel that there were really souls who have no faith, and who, through the abuse of grace, lost this precious treasure, the source of the only real and pure joys. He permitted my soul to be invaded by the thickest darkness, and that the thought of heaven, up until then so sweet to me, be no longer anything but the cause of struggle and torment. The trial was to last not a few days or a few weeks, it was not to be extinguished until the hour set by God Himself, and this hour has not yet come.[9]

Thérèse described traveling "through this dark tunnel" to reach a place like "a country that is covered in thick fog." It was there that she begged pardon for her fellow human beings' lack of faith. Describing herself in the third person while addressing divine presence, Thérèse resolved to "eat the bread of sorrow as long as You desire it; she does not wish to rise up from this table filled with bitterness at which poor sinners are eating until the day set by You." Instead of partaking in a joyful spiritual feast at the end of life, Thérèse thus underwent a trial of faith in which she saw herself making reparations for others' lack of faith. For as long as it took, Thérèse resigned herself to "eat this bread of trial at this table" while begging the heavenly world for mercy and pity.[10]

Having Supper with God: Issues of Faith and Devotion

Even as she ate at a banquet of sorrow, Thérèse recognized that her time in the shadows was a devotional offering and an act of love. At the end of life, such ambivalent imagery relating to dining, feasting, and spirituality can be extremely complex. One day I met a woman who was having great difficulty reconciling her existential pain and suffering with her devout religious beliefs. She openly acknowledged that she was "going to die" and she faced the reality of leaving several young children behind. She also expressed a strong spiritual perspective regarding what awaited her. As her mother explained, the woman

> *Loves her kids, and she loves God.*
> *God is really big in her life,*
> *And she wants to see Him.*
> *She says, "I'm going to go home and have supper with God."*
>
> *You live through God,*
> *And she will always be alive,*
> *To us, and to God.*

It Was Her Faith

Such images of feasting and facing the unknown also arose the day I met a very sweet family from Arkansas. In their narrative, they recounted the meaningful acts that their mother had performed with quiet modesty and great faith. These events had occurred many years ago, while the siblings were growing up in a small country town. Because the patient was extremely short of breath, her sisters told much of the story. When they had finished, the woman filled in the rest of the details. As I read the story aloud, one of the sisters movingly remarked, "I feel that our mother is smiling on us":

> *It Was Her Faith*
>
> *Our image is of our mother.*
> *She was very calm and patient.*

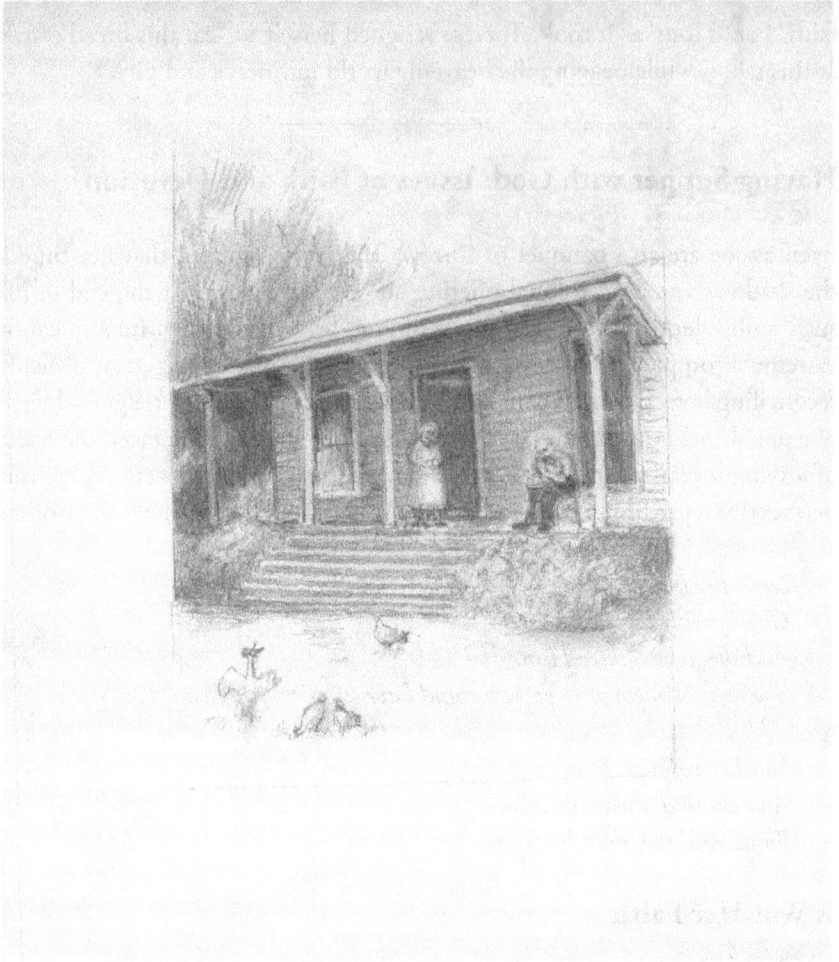

Figure 29: Lyn Smallwood, *It Was Her Faith*, 2015, graphite on white Arches paper

She was everything.
Her own mother died when she was only a girl,
So, she was raised more as an orphan.
Mother was the ultimate Christian.
She was little, and she was kind.

Our family is from Arkansas,
And we lived in the country.
When I was a very young girl,
A man came up to the porch.
We had a big white frame house,
And he came to the porch and walked up the stairs.
I can still see him, to this day.
He knocked, and Mother went up to the door.
He asked for something to eat.
He was an older man, with grayish white hair and a beard.
Mother went into the house and made him a plate of whatever we had—
Peas, cornbread—we had our dinner at lunch.
He ate, and she came back into the house,
And I asked her, "Why did you do this?"
And she said, "You never know if the Lord
Is sending one of his angels to test your faith.
It was an act of kindness."
I can't explain it.
It was her faith,
Knowing that God is real,
That He exists
And sends angels for different reasons.

There is another story that has travelled through our family,
About our brother.
When he was still a teenager he went into the Army.
It was World War II and he was on the front lines,
In one of the major battles in Belgium.
Oddly enough, he survived,
But no one heard from him for several months.
Mother didn't know if he was alive.

Our back porch was for shelling whatever came out of the garden.
Mother and Daddy were there with our sister.
It was the middle of the day,
And a rooster started crowing at the back door.
This was very unusual,
And Mother said, "Our son is coming home today,
And I'm going to cook a big dinner."
There were peas, and cornbread, and fried chicken,
And a coconut pie, which was our brother's favorite.
She was a great cook,
And she wouldn't let anyone eat until he got here.
Daddy just laughed.

Around the time when it got dark,
A car horn honked.
Mother said, "There he is."
And there he was.
He had hitched a ride with someone and come home.
It showed the trust Mother had in God.
She believed.
That rooster didn't tell her about our brother.
God told her.

I can't explain it.
It was her faith.

In the soft pencil drawing *It Was Her Faith* (Figure 29), Lyn Smallwood translates the family's narrative into a country genre scene. The viewer is positioned in front of the steps that lead to the broad front porch of the white frame farmhouse, where hens peck in the yard and a rooster crows alongside them. A diminutive woman stands before an open door and looks over at the softly glowing figure of an elderly man. The man quietly eats the plate of food that the woman has brought as an act of charity, while she gazes over at him with a shy smile.

This scene precedes the section of the narrative where the woman expressed prophetic knowledge of her son's return and she prepared a feast in anticipation of his arrival. Just as these acts were performed because "it was her faith" to do so, the story appears as a striking contrast *and* complement to Thérèse's visionary image of eating at the table of sorrow surrounded by people who lacked faith. Further resonating with Thérèse's themes, *It Was Her Faith* demonstrates how the simple, homely aspects of life can appear as sacred offerings. Such stories transform familiar perspectives of the world by presenting everyday reality as at once grounded and numinous. This story also incorporates a mystical element as it relates prophetic knowledge of future events. Even as the woman's husband dismissed the rooster's crowing as an omen, her deep faith enabled her to recognize aspects of life that remained hidden to others—in this case, giving the woman visionary knowledge that their son was alive and returning home despite having faced a deadly war battle in Belgium. Conjoining these themes, *It Was Her Faith* can be seen as an ambivalent narrative of blindness and vision, doubt and faith, the ordinary and the sacred.

The Veil of the Sky as the Obverse Side of Heaven

In her account of being led to the banquet of sorrow, Thérèse felt that the heaven world had been closed off as she passed through a tunnel and sat at a "table filled with bitterness." In the days that followed this dark mystical vision, Thérèse experienced pronounced physical pain as she faced her own grave illness. As she lamented, "My soul is exiled, heaven is closed for me, and on the earth's side it's all trial too."[11] Even as she endured such hardships, she expressed ambivalent feelings about the heaven world and its metaphorical equivalent on earth, the sky. As Thérèse reflected, "I admire the material heavens; the other is closed against me more and more. Then immediately I said to myself with great gentleness: Oh, certainly, it's really through love that I'm looking up at the sky; yes, it's through love for God, since everything that I do, my actions, my looks, everything, since my Offering, is done through love."[12]

From an early point, Thérèse perceived a profound connection between the earthly sky and the heavenly world. She recalled how, as a child walking home at night with her father, "I would gaze upon the *stars* that were twinkling ever so peacefully in the skies and the sight carried me away. There was especially one cluster of *golden pearls* that attracted my attention, and gave me great joy because they were in the form of a T. I pointed them out to Papa and told him my name was written in heaven." Thérèse asked her father to guide her footsteps as she looked upward, while throwing back her head and giving herself "over completely to the contemplation of the star-studded firmament!"[13]

In another youthful memory, Thérèse characterized the sky as a diaphanous veil that appeared as the "obverse side" of a "beautiful heaven." She recalled how, as children, she and her sister Céline would sit together during the evenings in the belvedere of their home where

> With enraptured gaze we beheld the white moon rising quietly behind the
> tall trees, the silvery rays it was casting upon sleeping nature, the bright stars
> twinkling in the deep skies, the light breath of the evening breeze making
> the snowy clouds float easily along; all this raised our souls to heaven, that
> beautiful heaven whose "obverse side" alone we were able to contemplate.[14]

In Thérèse's writings, the sky appears as a kind of diaphanous veil and as a
connective tissue that links the earthly and heavenly worlds. Similarly, people
at the end of life will reflect on the connections they perceive between the earth
and the heavens, images that are at once veiled and revealed in their stories of
the sky.

Stories of the Sky: Transitions Between Realms

One day I met a middle-aged man who described his experiences as both a
pilot and a skydiving paratrooper. He told me, "I guess you would say that, at
this point, I'm introspective." In his narrative, the inner and the outer worlds
converged in his vision of

A Clear Steel Blue

I became a pilot.
When you're flying,
You can get an image of God
From the beauty you see on a clear, steel blue day.

I was a paratrooper, and we would suit up and get into the aircraft.
When we arrived at the target
We would all stand up in a line by the open plane door.
The Jump Master would check our chutes,
And then he would give us the command,
Telling us when to jump.

Now, I'm seeing God as the Jump Master,
And I'm just waiting to be told,
When to jump

Figure 30: Lyn Smallwood, *Any Time I Look Up*, 2015, graphite on white Arches paper

Into the clear steel blue.

Drawing on his actual life experiences, the man envisioned a transitional zone that incorporated multiple states of being. Sometimes people at the end of life will describe the convergence of the natural and the supernatural realms through their perceptions of energetic presences that appear as sparkling golden and silver lights. Sometimes these etheric forms are associated with the sky, with its shifting clouds and evanescent light.

Any Time I Look Up

Closing the circle between first and last things, one day I visited with a lovely woman from Montana. While she had spent the bulk of her professional career as an obstetrical nurse, the woman now lay in bed at the very end of her life. As we visited together, she expressed her sense of inhabiting multiple worlds simultaneously. She recalled childhood experiences living in a spectacular natural landscape, imagery that became connected with her perception of the liminal spiritual presences she saw

Any Time I Look Up

My image is of clouds.
Mainly, they are free, and they are beautiful.
They come and they go.
You could look into the sky and find any gamut of emotion you find in life.
It's the images clouds provide.
I think they look a little different depending on where you're looking.

Looking up at the sky—
We did that a lot as kids,
And I think my kids did that, too.
We lived in the country, and we entertained ourselves a lot that way.

Any time I look up,
I can always find something that is a mood elevator,
Something that can bring me to a better place.
The clouds make me feel safe, and they rejuvenate me.

The clouds definitely have a spiritual significance.
They are a good way to fill the void in your thoughts.
The clouds are a close outer periphery
Of what makes me feel safe and secure.

Since I've been here, in Palliative Care at M.D. Anderson,
About six times a day,
I see flickers, like the edges of a silhouette.
It's like smoky, white, foggy edges.
They're very comforting.
I've noticed them,
And it's like a presentation of someone saying:
Hello, I'm here, and all is well.
I also noticed them when I was working as an obstetrical nurse,
The flickers of silhouettes,
Coming and going.

They present just like clouds do.
They're there, and then, they're not there.

Blurring the boundaries between worlds, the woman's artwork unites the domains of obstetrics and palliative care as it tells a story of beginnings and ends, of life and death. As I began reading her narrative aloud, the woman took my hand in hers. Despite her repeated protests that she was never a writer—and that she had never been good at producing compositions in school—she quickly recognized her own voice in this remarkable story. As she listened, she appeared to be almost radiant as she heard the beauty of her narrative.

With its themes of transience and evanescence, Lyn Smallwood's soft pencil drawing *Any Time I Look Up* (Figure 30) draws on transitional images of the sky to locate subtle spiritual presences within the familiar realm of everyday life. The artwork utilizes the motif of the transparent windowpane to create an ambivalent framing mechanism. Depicting the scene that the woman described, the image features the luminous traces of a diaphanous figure whose translucent silhouette closely resembles the cloud formations that appear just outside the window. This enigmatic figure stands within the solid inner walls of the woman's hospital room, yet its ethereal form resonates with the soft clouds that float loosely overhead.

Such visionary themes arose the day I visited with a middle-aged man who was very weak and frail; only his face showed above the edge of the heavy white hospital blanket. While he was short of breath and only had the strength to speak in whispers, the man was acutely aware of the world around him. Knowing that our visit would be very brief, I drew a chair up to his bedside and leaned in closely to catch his words. As he spoke, I was struck by the way in which his tone was at once matter-of-fact yet reverential as he shared his image of

A Warm, Bright Light

My image is of a warm, bright light.
I can see it.
It looks fluorescent.
It's about as close as between you and me.
I've seen it all my life.
That bright light makes me feel warm and peaceful.

Throughout the visit, we were sitting about eighteen inches away from one another. As the man described his vision of a warm bright light that was as present and close by as I was, his words evoked a suggestive convergence of the existential and the spiritual realms. Such narratives provide new ways to contemplate subjects that are simultaneously coming into form and going out of form within the framework of a single story.

The Picture That Cannot Be Pictured: Vision and Blindness in the Aniconic Icon

While *A Warm, Bright Light* and *Any Time I Look Up* relate a sense of seeing what cannot ordinarily be seen, sometimes people will emphasize the invisibility of their image of the sacred. Both Thérèse's writings and end-of-life narratives can express such a saying of unsaying—and with it, a sense of the absence of presence and the holding of the unholdable. If I were to phrase this in technical terms, I would say that we were encountering the aniconic icon—a paradoxical figure that evokes a simultaneous sense of affirmation and negation as it asserts and denies the visibility of its own presence.

One day I met a very elderly man from Guatemala who was about to leave for hospice care. When I asked him if there was an image in his mind of something that was significant for him, the man engaged very simple language to express an extremely complex idea—namely, the concept of a divinity whose presence was simultaneously affirmed and denied within the framework of his imagery. Drawing on a familiar metaphor, the man candidly stated:

Nobody Ever Took a Picture

The most important thing in my mind is God.
If they wanted to put another image in my mind,
I wouldn't let them.
Nobody on earth ever took a picture of God.
No one in this world could make an image of God.

When I think of God,
I feel secure, and I feel hope.
When I read the word of God,
Everything is there.
God is God.

In this narrative, the man described the paradox of the picture that cannot be pictured. As he related his conception of the sacred, he expressed a simultaneous sense of giving and withholding. Such narratives evoke an image that simultaneously asserts and denies the power of its own presence. These paradoxical themes also resonate with Thérèse's images of presence and absence, and her insistence on her own insignificance. As she told her sister Pauline: "No, I'm not a saint; I've never performed the actions of a saint. I'm a very little soul upon whom God has bestowed graces; that's what I am." Thérèse then remarked: "I have lights only to see my little nothingness. This does me more good than all the lights on the faith."[15] In having lights to see only her "little nothingness," Thérèse expressed not only her innate humility, but the assertion of a negation—the greatness of littleness that holds the nothing that is potentially everything.

With Empty Hands: The Overflowing Presence of Absence

Thérèse was a master at holding the unholdable. Just as the torn veil appears as an image that holds what cannot otherwise be held, while she was still quite young, Thérèse envisioned the offering of love and self-overcoming that she would make at the very end of her life. Addressing divinity, Thérèse reflected that, "In the evening of this life, I shall appear before You with empty hands."[16] Both literally and symbolically, Thérèse's expressive gesture embodies the fullness of emptiness as she pictured the absence that can encompass and contain all things. Returning to these themes at the end of her life, Thérèse told her superior that everything she had was for others, and that "I hold nothing in my hands."[17] In emphasizing her empty hands and her intrinsic littleness in "becoming nothing," Thérèse could potentially become everything—that is, she could become all things by becoming nothing, and she could become nothing by humbly becoming all things. Through her paradoxical image of empty hands, Thérèse could evoke the delicacy, fragility, and finite nature of her own humanity in all of its limitations, while simultaneously recognizing that, within these very finite qualities lay the becoming of nothing that held the infinite possibility of becoming everything, and the death of death that represents another form of life itself.

Sometimes caring for people at the end of life similarly entails attention to the subtle vocabulary that arises when individuals speak in a language of silence, when they communicate through overflowing gestures made with empty hands. One day I met the family of an extremely elderly man who was on the threshold of actively dying, and who would ultimately pass away later that evening. While visiting with this family, I learned that the man was a Holocaust survivor, and that his childhood experiences growing up in Eastern Europe had deeply shaped his personal character and how he lived his life. The man could no longer speak, and he drifted in and out of consciousness while we created a tribute to him. When I told the family that the story was complete and I prepared to read it aloud, the man opened his eyes, looked directly into my eyes, and beckoned me to his side. I returned his gaze and introduced myself. He held out his left hand, which I took in my right hand as I read the artwork. The man followed along closely, and he smiled and even laughed at one point. When I had finished reading, the man squeezed my hand, and then, with his right index finger he made a sweeping circular gesture around the room, indicating how much he loved his family and how much he valued each of them.

I have never forgotten the tenderness of this encounter or the inclusive power of the man's circular gesture. During this visit the man's empty hands overflowed with meaning as he spoke eloquently in a language of silence. Just as he gave me a new perspective on holding the unholdable, I knew, once again, that I was sitting in the presence of a rose from two gardens.

Notes

1. Quoted in *Story of a Soul*, 54-55.
2. Quoted in *Story of a Soul*, 74–75.
3. Quoted in *St. Thérèse of Lisieux*, 88.
4. On these themes, see Mary Frohlich, "The 'Thirst of Jesus' in the Vocations of Mother Teresa and Thérèse of Lisieux," *New Theology Review* 21, no. 4 (November 2008), 70–77. Frohlich observes that the sense of "interior darkness" that Mother Teresa of Calcutta and Thérèse of Lisieux experienced relate to a venerable Christian mystical tradition of feeling profound hunger and thirst for the infinite love of God. Within and beyond their examples, mystical darkness is seen as the mark of a finite being longing for communion with the infinite. I am grateful to Gregory Perron for bringing this article to my attention.
5. Quoted in *St. Thérèse of Lisieux*, 113.
6. Quoted in *Story of a Soul*, 268–71.
7. See the definition of "ecstasy" in *Webster's Seventh New Collegiate Dictionary*, 262.
8. Quoted in *Story of a Soul*, 210.
9. Quoted in *Story of a Soul*, 211–12.
10. Quoted in *Story of a Soul*, 211–12.
11. Quoted in *St. Thérèse of Lisieux*, 68. On these themes, see Nevin, *The Last Years of Saint Thérèse*.
12. Quoted in *St. Thérèse of Lisieux*, 141.
13. Quoted in *Story of a Soul*, 42–43.
14. Quoted in *Story of a Soul*, 103. As John Clarke notes, Thérèse is referencing Alfred Besse de Larzes's poem *L'envers du Ciel* (1880).
15. Quoted in *St. Thérèse of Lisieux*, 143, 148.
16. Quoted in *Story of a Soul*, 277. Thérèse also expressed these words in her Act of Oblation, the statement of spiritual devotion and surrender that she made on June 9, 1895.
17. Quoted in *St. Thérèse of Lisieux*, 91.

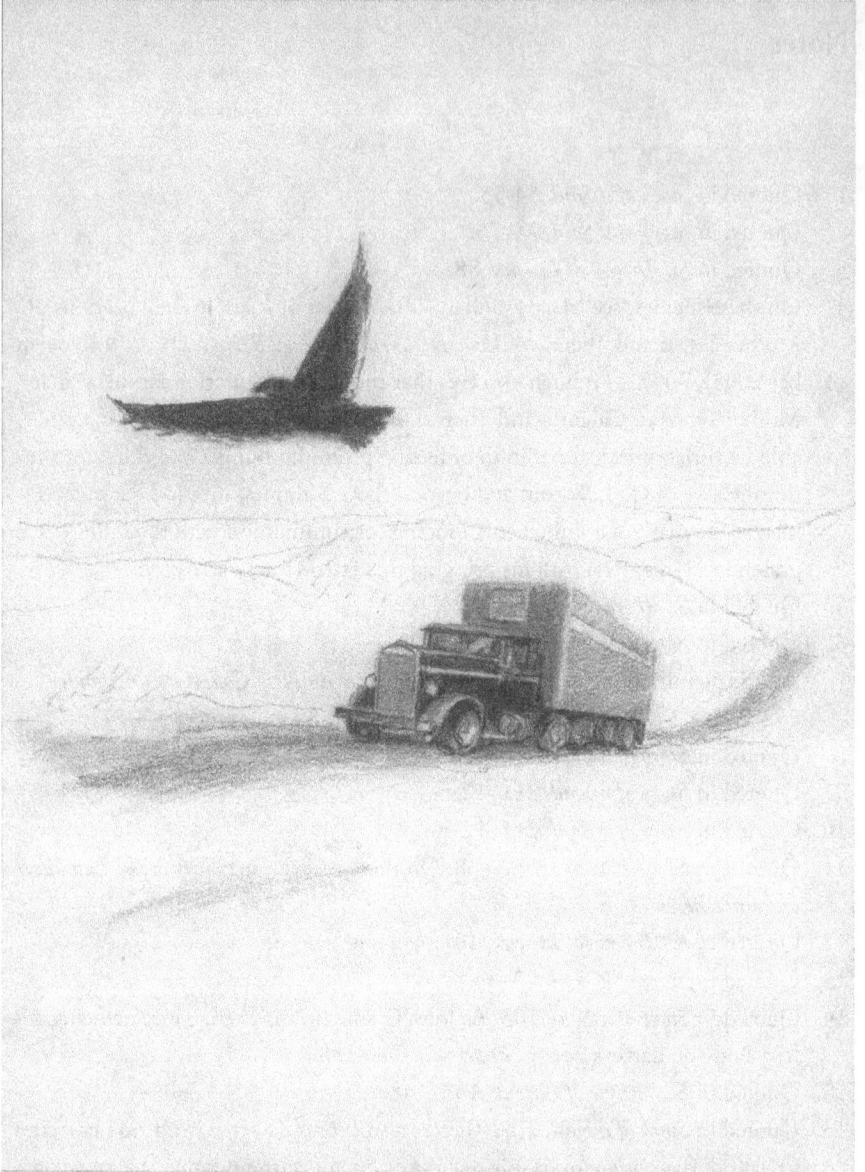

Figure 31: Lyn Smallwood, *The Black Bird*, 2020, graphite on white Strathmore drawing paper

Chapter Eight

The Connection is Love:
Facing Death and Seeing Life

The Black Bird: Connections Between Worlds

One day I visited with a Mexican family who told an extraordinary story about their traditions. The patient was an older man who suffered from an extremely aggressive form of cancer. He had been admitted to the Acute Palliative Care Unit earlier that day for pain control. The man only spoke Spanish, so his adult daughter served as his translator as he told a striking story of

The Black Bird

My dad has always been a truck driver.
All his life, it's been his job and his passion.
And, it's a family heritage.
All of his brothers were truck drivers.
It's in the family.
He and his brothers would all get together and talk about things.
One of the relatives would see something bad on the road,
And they would alert my dad
And tell him to be careful.

The truck my dad drove was called "The Black Bird."
It was named after my uncle, who was my dad's oldest brother.
The black bird is a dark, massive bird with bright wings.
It's a wild bird, and it flies very fast.
They named the truck after my dad's brother,
Who was also dark and very fast,

Just like the bird.

His brother died of cancer,
And so did many of the male relatives.
It's the same type of cancer my father has.
This is also the family heritage.
This is also part of their tradition.

My dad has no spiritual fears.
He is in peace with God.
Yesterday morning my dad told me
He saw his brothers and other male relatives in the room.
He was asleep, and they were touching him,
And he woke up.
When he woke up he asked my mom,
"Where are all the people in the room?"
And my mom was like, "What people?"
My dad said his brothers were touching him as he woke up.

That's how he knows he's ready
To go to heaven.

This story is at once grounded and soaring, harrowing and uplifting. Through the highs and the lows of life and death, the family maintained a powerful sense of connection. This became especially poignant as the man described how all of the male relatives stuck together through difficult times, both during their lifetimes and thereafter, and how they reappeared as he prepared to make yet another journey.

In Lyn Smallwood's pencil illustration (Figure 31), a man drives a massive dark truck through the steep hilly roads of Mexico while a large black bird with outstretched wings circles overhead. The detailed forms of the truck and the bird evoke the man's older brother and their shared family history. Just as the image is stark and iconic, it raises suggestive questions concerning whether we are witnessing a scene from life or from a dream. With its vivid details of the truck, the brothers, the bird, and the flight, *The Black Bird* encompasses the relations between matter and spirit, joining and loss, doubling and unification. By engaging these themes, the story emphasizes the bonds that exist both within and beyond familiar conceptions of time and being.

Like many end-of-life narratives, this story evokes the ways in which people envision otherwise unseen presences as they approach death.[1] In this chapter, I share the stories of people who describe seeing, sensing, touching, and recognizing the subtle presences of those who have passed on. While these subjects may seem abstract and metaphysical, the narratives are grounded, intimate, and very human. As individuals describe meeting their loved ones in dreams and transient visions, they engage with these figures in ways that are both ordinary and extraordinary. As a result, the stories convey a doubled sense of the familiar and the numinous. As though poised in a state of contingency, the artworks offer unique perspectives on the possibilities that lie at the boundaries of life itself. Despite the controversial status of such narratives in end-of-life care, the stories can be extremely powerful not only for the people who tell them, but also for all of us. Again and again the artworks express the insight that, when facing death, we see life.

We Don't Think About Death Enough: Thérèse on the End of Life

Thérèse of Lisieux also reflected on the ways in which the experiences of birth and death, life and the afterlife, are connected through the power of love. Thérèse was well aware of the challenges associated with integrating conceptions of death into life itself. Prior to joining the convent, Thérèse experienced the pleasures and luxuries of life, yet she was critical of friends whom she felt were "too worldly; they knew too well how to ally the joys of this earth to the service of God. They didn't think about *death* enough, and yet *death* had paid its visit to a great number of souls whom I knew, the young, the rich, the happy!" While openly acknowledging the presence of death, Thérèse cared for the world around her. She recalled how, as a schoolgirl, she tended to nature's most vulnerable creatures: "I had invented a game which pleased me, and it was to bury the poor little birds we found dead under the trees. Many of the students wanted to help me, and so our cemetery became very beautiful, planted with trees and flowers in proportion to the size of our little feathered friends."[2] From these early gestures of compassion to later attending fellow nuns as they passed away, to her ultimate confrontation with her own premature death, Thérèse's life reflects an ongoing dialogue between the mortal and the eternal, the human and the mystical.

As Thérèse keenly observed, too often people don't know how to respond to those who are dying or to those who have passed on. My experiences have shown me that, when facing the end of life, it's as though people are looking at broken wrenches, blunt nails, and blankets with holes in them—it's as though individuals are looking at things they don't know what to do with, and they often feel a sense of shame or anxiety. Sometimes fear comes in as people stand at the graveside and see their loved one in the casket and watch as the person is put into the ground. Such experiences can trigger consciousness of one's own mortality, as people realize that they may be the next in line to go. For various reasons, individuals can be afraid to be happy when someone passes on, and this can create great difficulty in honoring the emotional aspect of the experience. Yet when individuals have visions of their loved ones who have passed on, they often feel the power of love and a strong sense of accompaniment. When this occurs, people can walk a well-worn road, yet it feels soothing, and even like velvet.

End-of-life artworks will similarly engage the presence of transient and ineffable subjects that simultaneously crystalize and dissolve before our eyes. Such stories take us deep into the terrain of secrets and mysteries—including both their hiddenness and their uncovering. In this context, the word "crypt" is particularly suggestive. Derived from the Greek *kryptos*, the term relates to that which is hidden. The word is also akin to the Old Norse *hreysar*, which signifies a "heap of stones." As a noun, a crypt signifies "a chamber (as a vault) wholly or partly underground." As an adjective, the cryptic denotes subjects that are secret, enigmatic, mysterious, obscure, unrecognized, or encoded.[3] Just as a crypt designates a subterranean location where bodies are buried, the exposed presence of the stones represents a marker of concealment *and* of disclosure. As such, the crypt evokes the ambivalent presence of absence, just as it stands as a material yet occult sign of hiding and showing, of the seen and the unseen. The crypt is thus a nondual location, a repository that holds the secrets of both the deaths and the lives that are revealed and concealed in a common place of presence.[4]

Resonating with these themes, toward the end of her life Thérèse was shown a photograph of herself, to which she replied, "Yes, but … this is the envelope; when will we see the letter? Oh! how I want to see the letter!"[5] Thérèse's suggestive statement engages the relations between the seen and the unseen, the external appearance of familiar forms and the intrinsic presence of inner life. As we reflect on these subjects, we too encounter the relations between the empirical and the visionary, the domain of secrets and the possibility of their uncovering.

Close at Hand: Feeling the Presences of Those Who Are No Longer Here

Shortly after I began doing this work, I met a quiet woman who was a retired nurse. When I asked her about her imagery, the woman immediately told me about her mother. As we visited, her familiar images formed the basis of a visionary artwork:

There She Is

I've always thought about my mother,
Where she is, and how she's doing.
My mother passed away many years ago,
But I carry her driver's license in my purse,
To have a clear portrait of her.

I don't normally talk about her.
But after she passed, I would think of her,
And I could see her standing there.
Then she would disappear.

I keep her picture with me, all the time.
We were like sisters.

Such stories offer unique perspectives on how those who are no longer here may be present in other ways. Much like the writings of Thérèse, this narrative evokes the sense that the numinous is readily accessible and close at hand. Clothed in a language of simplicity and directness, the story feels both ordinary and extraordinary. As we read such narratives, we too may feel an expanded sense of presence.

Another woman told me a moving story about her daughter. Before I entered this room, the staff had described the woman as being difficult and having fluctuating states of mind, as she would go from complaining about the food one moment to speaking of seeing her deceased daughter the next. Yet throughout our visit, the woman spoke lucidly. I barely had time to finish inscribing her narrative when the ambulance attendants arrived to discharge the woman to home hospice care. She then remarked that it was "interesting timing" that she had just enough time to tell me about her daughter:

She's My Whole Life

My image is of my daughter.
She lived a very short life—
She was murdered.
But, every mother in the world should have a daughter like that.

I know she's waiting for me in heaven.
I tell her I'm not ready to be with her yet,
But I see her and talk to her every day of my life.
She's my whole life.

This story sheds light on an ambivalent aspect of end-of-life experience. Despite reporting positive encounters with her deceased daughter, the woman still feared her own death and she was afraid to pass on. Notwithstanding the burden of her advanced illness, she had great difficulty letting go, and she refused to tell the staff why she was not yet ready to be with her daughter. When other members of the team approached her on this subject, the woman would turn her head to one side on the pillow and look away, and this made for an extremely prolonged end-of-life transition.

On another day I visited with a family whom the team characterized as "high distress." While two of the adult children were very tearful, I was surprised by what I found when I entered the room. The patient was an older man who was nonresponsive and rapidly declining, but he was not yet actively dying. Throughout our visit, the man was smiling and reaching his arms up high, and he had an expression of radiant joy on his face. While he could no longer speak, his youngest son told me that his father was

Having visions and reaching out to people.
For the past day or so, he's been reaching out and pulling up.
It's like he's pulling on a rope.
I was there when our mother passed away,
And she did the same thing.
I think his life is fulfilled.
I think he's being called back home.

In the hospital, you never know what you will find on the other side of a patient's closed door. Each situation is unique, and humility is key. Sometimes people's spiritual experiences are elusive and ambiguous, while at other times, people relate very clear and concrete visions of their metaphysical encounters. Whatever form the stories take, the narratives can serve as valued points of continuity between worlds.

Just Trust Me: The Eyes of Jesus

One day I visited with the son of an older woman who was rapidly becoming disoriented. When I asked him to tell me about his mother, the man recalled a near-death experience she had a few years before:

Just Trust Me: The Eyes of Jesus

A few years ago, my mother and I were attending a birthday party.
Her car was giving her difficulties,
And I said, "You drive my truck, and I'll drive your car."
We were on the feeder road.
As I looked at the truck in my rear view mirror,
I saw my mother getting struck broadside at ninety miles per hour,
And getting flipped over, four times.

The pickup truck was crushed, and the engine was smoking.
I ran over and said, "Mama, are you alright?"
She said, "Come and get me out of this truck before it blows up."
I carried her out and laid her down.
She suffered from broken pelvic bones,
But since then, with therapy, she's been able to walk again.

When the accident happened,
Jesus was already with her, in the truck.
When she got hit, she spoke with Jesus, in that pickup truck.
Jesus told her, "Put your hands on the roof of the truck,
And we're going to roll."
After the third roll He said, "We're going to roll one more time."
He also said, "Just trust me."
My mother said that His eyes were the only thing that appeared,
And that when He was there,
The truck lit up as a huge light.

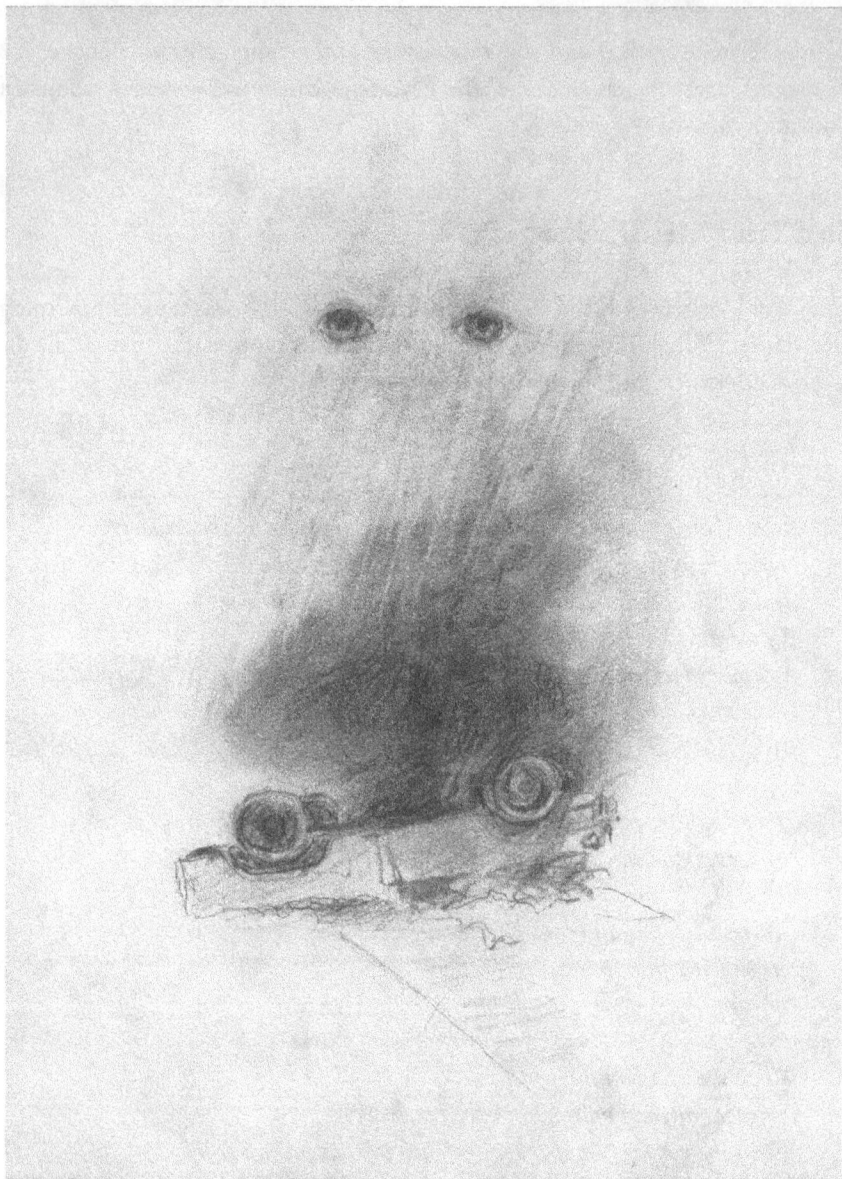

Figure 32: Lyn Smallwood, *The Eyes of Jesus*, 2021, graphite on white Strathmore drawing paper

In this story of trauma and grace, a woman describes seeing the radiant eyes of Jesus amidst the devastation of a car crash. Mirroring these themes, the lower two-thirds of Lyn Smallwood's illustration (Figure 32) displays a horrific car wreck. Thick black smoke issues from the damaged body of a pickup truck that lies flipped over on a highway. In the upper register of the composition, the luminous eyes of a holy figure whom the woman identified as Jesus look down tenderly. The eyes are filled with both power and compassion as they gaze into the place where the swirling dark smoke of the wreck meets a rising stream of white light.

Thérèse similarly described seeing the luminous eyes of Jesus looking down at her as she crossed through a dark tunnel. In September of 1890, shortly before her profession of vows, Thérèse related a scene in which Jesus led her through "a tunnel where I see nothing but a half-veiled light, the brightness shining from the eyes of Jesus looking down."[6] Both passages describe transitional spaces in which the eyes of Jesus illuminate otherwise darkened scenes. As Thérèse and the woman at the end of life described their experiences, they expressed a simultaneous sense of immersion in—and transcendence of—the world around them.

From the Prenatal to the Postmortem Realms: Multi-Generational Love Stories

A different expression of the continuity of presence arises when people anticipate their own passing and they envision an ongoing relationship with those who are still here. One day I met an older woman who lived a very difficult life, having raised several of her grandchildren on her own. Now facing the end of her life, the woman was imagining a continuing relationship with her family after she passed away:

That's My Soul

My image is of an angel.
That's my soul.
That's my serenity.
I want my family to know that
I have wisdom to give,
No matter where I am.

Just as she visualized her soul as an angel, the woman imagined an ongoing relationship that spanned multiple realms of being. After I read her artwork aloud, I remarked that the family could always call on this woman, no matter where she was, to which she immediately replied: "Absolutely!"

On another day, I visited with a woman whose brother lay dying. After chatting for a few minutes, the woman informed me:

About a week ago,
My brother told me Mom was coming for him.
So, he knows.
My brother told me—and God told me—that he's ready,
And he's at peace.
This lets me be at peace, as well.

The woman then shared a family history in which, prior to their deaths, the men in the family searched for—and found—their deceased mothers. The woman recalled her father's passing:

About a week before he passed,
My father said he was looking for his mom,
And that my grandfather was going to show him where she was.
When we talked that time, he was still looking for his mom,
And he had that worried and distracted look.
So, it would not have been a peaceful passing.
My father had amputations from diabetes,
And he was dying of gangrene.

The last time I spoke to my father,
It was just before he passed.
I asked him if he was ready to die.
I needed to know, in order to be at peace.
He smiled at me and he said,
"I found Mom."

Shortly after this conversation, the older man passed away peacefully, and the woman never forgot the story. Similar themes arose as her brother now faced the end of his life. Even as the woman anticipated this loss with some difficulty, she was greatly comforted that both her father and her brother expressed the same message: "I found Mom."

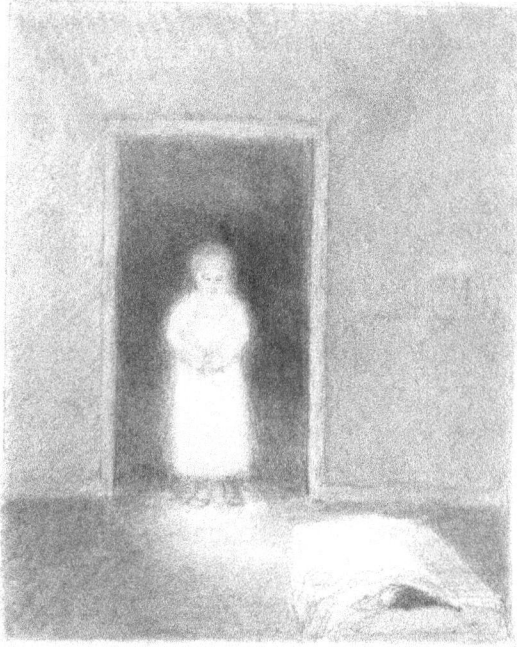

Figure 33: Lyn Smallwood, *So Bright*, 2014, graphite on white Arches paper

So Bright

Sometimes family stories will extend in multiple directions at once as the narratives reference people who are currently living, people who are no longer here, and people who are not yet here—that is, babies who are expected but who have yet to be born. One afternoon a young woman told an extraordinary story of such intergenerational connections. Notably, this was a visit that almost didn't occur, as the woman was an off-service lymphoma patient who happened to be on the Acute Palliative Care Unit while awaiting a stem cell transplant. For this reason, she was the last patient I saw at the end of a long day. As she and I reflected on this later, we were both so glad that the visit unfolded, as we felt it was a gift for both of us.

When I asked the woman what she loved to do, she described singing in the choir. She particularly loved the classical music that was performed in Latin and in other European languages. As she said, "There's just something about it. It feels very empowering. It makes you feel like you are somewhere else, like all your problems have gone away. It takes you somewhere peaceful, quiet and calm." When I asked her to describe the place where the music took her, she started to talk about a place of miracles, and how the birth of her youngest daughter was like a miracle to her:

So Bright

My youngest daughter is my miracle baby.
I was diagnosed with lymphoma when I was a few months pregnant.
I told the doctors that I would wait to take the chemo
Until after I had my daughter,
And they said no, that if I waited, I'd be dead by then.
The doctor told me I had to have an abortion because of the chemo,
And I said, "No, I'm sorry. I don't believe in that.
If God gave her to me, it has to be for a reason."
I found a doctor here at M.D. Anderson who was willing to work with me,
Who explained all the risks.
And there I was, with my big belly, taking chemo.
Today, my daughter is healthy, and she is so smart.

So many miracles have occurred in my life.
When I was first pregnant with her,
One time, I was really, really sick.

I was running a high fever.
I couldn't even talk or move.
I was lying in bed drenched in sweat.
My great-grandmother was on her deathbed,
And everyone had gone to the hospital,
So I couldn't call anyone.
I tried to get up to get a glass of water
And I just fell back down.

Then I told God,
If it's my time, I give myself to you.
I'm in your arms.
Just remember, I have my family.
But I give myself to you.

Then I saw someone standing in the doorway.
I asked, "Who is there?"
But no one answered.
I asked if someone had come home from the hospital.
Again, no one answered.
Then I looked more closely,
And I could see a presence.
It was so bright.
I heard a voice say,
"You're going to be okay. Don't worry."
And I asked, "Grandma, is that you?"
And then the phone rang, and I grabbed it.
It was my mother calling,
She said, "Your great-grandmother has just passed away."
I turned around and looked again
And she wasn't there.
But it was such a huge miracle, and a blessing.

I was really sick, and the next day I went to the hospital.
At the hospital, they said I was having a miscarriage,
And that I could have died.
At the time, I didn't even know I was pregnant.
But then, when they told me,
I knew that, when my great-grandmother said,

"You're going to be okay,"
That she was talking about both of us.

In Lyn Smallwood's drawing, *So Bright* (Figure 33), a young woman lies in bed struggling with severe illness. Standing in an otherwise darkened doorway, the glowing presence of the woman's great-grandmother appears in spirit form as an extremely bright light. While framed in this dark space, the great-grandmother casts a luminous shadow on the floor, projecting a band of light that connects her upright standing form to the horizontal figure of the young woman lying in the bed. The older woman looks down at her great-granddaughter, and their eyes meet in a tender exchange of love and recognition. On multiple levels, this drawing conjoins clarity and softness through modulated passages of darkness and light. While one woman is older and the other is younger, a subtle resemblance is apparent in their facial features, as both women are poised at the transitions of life and death and new life.

After I read the story aloud, the woman smiled and cried. She told me that she wants the story to be shared with others, and she tells it to everyone because

It Gives People Hope

I like to tell this story,
Especially to other patients,
To people who are depressed, and waiting to die,
People who have no hope.
You can see them light up and get stronger
When they hear the story.

Yes, I like to tell this story.
These are the types of things you hear about from other people,
But when you go through it yourself,
That's when you believe it.

Just as the boundaries that separate and conjoin the realms of the dying, the dead, and the living can become quite fluid, expanded conceptions of life can emerge within these transcendent spaces. By engaging the relations between the prenatal and the postmortem realms, this story raises provocative questions such as: Who are the dead, and who are the living? What can it mean to be in the presence of a living presence? Is the woman's great-grandmother dead or living—or potentially, both at once? Who gets to say? How do we determine the ontological status of such subjects, and how do we find language to account for such experiences?

The Controversial Status of End-of-Life Visions

In his classic study of the psychology of religion, *The Varieties of Religious Experience* (1902), the philosopher William James identified four characteristics associated with mystical experience. They include a sense of ineffability, transiency, passivity, and a noetic quality. In this volume, James compiled numerous primary accounts of people's mystical experiences. One of the recurrent features of the narratives concerns the ways in which love helps to transform ineffable experiences into recognizable presences, even as these presences often remain subtle and invisible.[7]

While a comprehensive discussion of these complex subjects lies beyond the scope of this volume, here I will note that, while mystical experiences represent familiar topics in end-of-life care, they also remain the subject of much debate. Within the extensive literature on these topics, end-of-life visions and near-death experiences are sometimes celebrated as meaningful and valuable, and sometimes they are dismissed as false or hallucinatory.[8] Whether expressed as a dream or a sensation or a vision, when people relate their subtle spiritual experiences, the encounters can risk being devalued or written off as delusional, even as they may hold great meaning for the people involved.

As the sociologist Allan Kellehear notes, the phenomena of spirit visions and end-of-life visitations are difficult to discuss openly. In part, this is due to the ways in which modern cultural discourses have become polarized between the proponents of these events and skeptics who dismiss them as hallucinatory and pathological. While such well-established polemics tend to produce the predictably fraught binary responses of esoteric mysticism and scientific rationalism, Kellehear advocates that emphasis be placed instead on the social meanings that these events can hold, and the personal value they can inspire for those who experience them.[9] As he notes, there is a pressing need to incorporate such discussions into how we approach the end of life, especially when we encounter extraordinary states of consciousness that are too often dismissed. For these reasons, when people at the end of life, or those who have experienced bereavement, describe "perceptions of objects or experiences that seem to have 'no objective reality,'"[10] we would do well to listen respectfully and consider the ways in which these subjects may hold great value for the person and those around them.

One day I met a woman whom the team described as being confused and delusional, primarily because she described speaking with imaginary presences. The patient was an elderly woman on high-flow oxygen. Her husband of many decades sat devotedly at her bedside. During our visit the woman was short of breath, yet she was lucid and oriented to the world around her. As the woman described the care she received on so many levels, her husband commented on the woman's spiritual experiences:

> *As soon as we got here,*
> *I knew she felt the Spirit.*
> *She was crying.*
> *And, I felt it, too.*
> *We're married for more than fifty years,*
> *And, I knew.*

While some individuals recognize the ways in which such metaphysical narratives can be uplifting and transformative, others may respond in ways that are dismissive and marginalizing. If, in a clinical context, a person says that they can see, hear, speak with, or touch a deceased loved one, then that individual risks being characterized as confused, irrational, or otherwise not fully oriented. Because this phenomenon cannot be reproduced or experienced by others, it cannot be independently or objectively verified, as standards of empirical validity are being applied (sometimes explicitly, sometimes implicitly) to subtle spiritual experiences. So much seems to depend on what any given person can imagine, accommodate, or identify with. These subjects are complex. While there is clear value in preserving mechanisms to evaluate lucidity, rationality, and cognitive acuity, it is also important to keep in mind that objectivity and subjectivity are dialectical constructs, and that both are intrinsic to human consciousness.

This discussion raises related questions concerning: Whose voices are being heard, and whose perspectives are being honored, at the end of life? Within the clinical context, whose job is it to sit and listen as people tell their stories? While these activities clearly fall within the scope of caregiving, various factors can contribute to the challenges associated with integrating these subjects into end of life care. In so many ways, the end of life is the undoing of a human life, and attending people at this time can be difficult and exhausting. The boundaries that separate *and* connect individuals are not always sharply drawn and they can become permeable. At the personal level, caregivers can feel overwhelmed and exhausted by practical and emotional demands, particularly as they grapple with their own sense of grief, fear, loss, or sadness. Within the medical context, palliative care represents a relatively new and sometimes controversial field of medicine. There simply is not a long history of having a critical mass of dying people assembled within an institutional setting that emphasizes end-of-life care rather than an aggressive stance toward cure. While medical professionals are accustomed to addressing pain and suffering, for various reasons they can be reluctant to engage questions of spirituality. While individuals often speak movingly of the valuable support that spirituality offers at the end of life, these themes can be very difficult to translate into a clinical context.[11] For all of these reasons, the services of an interdisciplinary palliative care team can be particularly valuable, as counselors, chaplains, and artists can all play instrumental roles in providing care and support during this transitional time. Above all, my work has shown me the value of approaching these sensitive issues from a patient-centered point of view. When I speak with people, our conversations tend to focus on what matters most in their lives, and how they imagine what comes next. A sense of fluidity often arises as people envision continuities of presence and they describe subtle connections between worlds.

Going Behind the Veil, Again: Visionary Encounters With Sacred Presences

One of Thérèse's most striking mystical experiences arose in a dream that occurred approximately a year and a half before her death. When recalling the dream, Thérèse described a scene in which she encountered three veiled Carmelite nuns, one of whom was identified as Anne de Lobera (Ana de Jesús, 1545–1621). A contemporary of Saint Teresa of Ávila (1515–1582), Anne de Lobera founded the Carmel in France during the early seventeenth century. Prior to the dream, Thérèse admitted that she had not thought of this figure unless she was mentioned by others. Yet Thérèse was struck by the love that this nun directed toward her. Thérèse's account deserves to be quoted at length:

> At the first glimmerings of dawn I was (in a dream) in a kind of gallery and there were several other persons, but they were at a distance. Our Mother was alone near me. Suddenly, without seeing how they had entered, I saw three Carmelites dressed in their mantles and long veils. It appeared to me they were coming for our Mother, but what I did understand clearly was that they

came from heaven. In the depths of my heart I cried out: "Oh! How happy I would be if I could see the face of one of these Carmelites!" Then, as though my prayer were heard by her, the tallest of the saints advanced toward me; immediately I fell to my knees. Oh! what happiness! the Carmelite *raised her veil or rather she raised it and covered me with it*. Without the least hesitation, I recognized *Venerable Anne of Jesus*, Foundress of the Carmel in France. Her face was beautiful but with an immaterial beauty. No ray escaped from it and still, in spite of the veil which covered us both, I saw this heavenly face suffused with an unspeakably gentle light, a light it didn't receive from without but was produced from within.

Thérèse then described her conversation with this holy figure:

Seeing myself so tenderly loved, I dared to pronounce these words: "O Mother! I beg you, tell me whether God will leave me for a long time on earth. Will He come soon to get me?" Smiling tenderly, the saint whispered: "*Yes, soon, soon, I promise you.*" I added: "Mother, tell me further if God is not asking something more of me than my poor little actions and desires. Is He content with me?" The saint's face took on an expression *incomparably more tender* than the first time she spoke to me. Her look and her caresses were the sweetest of answers. However, she said to me: "God asks no other thing from you. He is content, very content!" After again embracing me with more love than the tenderest of mothers has ever given to her child, I saw her leave. My heart was filled with joy, and then I remembered my Sisters, and I wanted to ask her some favors for them, but alas, I awoke![12]

In this passage, Thérèse described the paradox of lifting a veil to go behind a veil. Anne de Lobera's veil can be seen not only as part of the habit of the Carmelite nun, but also as a kind of threshold plane, a permeable boundary that marked a passageway for visionary experience. While beneath the veil, Thérèse was able to see in a subtle light, and she could feel great love as she gained extraordinary knowledge. Put another way, Thérèse's mystical encounter behind the veil encompassed the presences of both the envelope and the letter. After this experience, Thérèse observed that the dream affirmed that "there was a *heaven* and that this *heaven* is peopled with souls who actually love me, who consider me their child."[13] For Thérèse, the mystical dream confirmed the existence of a heaven world filled with love and with the ongoing presence of continuing life.

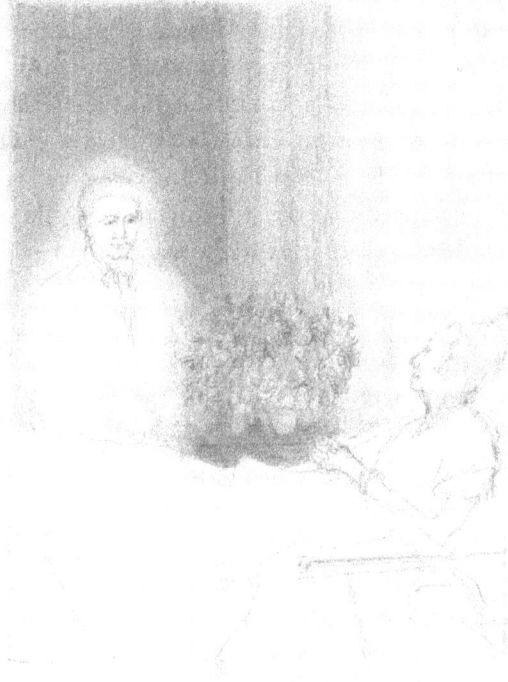

Figure 34: Lyn Smallwood, *And That Completes the Story*, 2015, graphite on white Arches paper

And That Completes the Story: Facing Death and Seeing Life

Despite the pervasive sense of uncertainty, shame, anxiety, and fear that our culture often associates with death, the writings of Thérèse of Lisieux and the poetic narratives of people at the end of life can shed important light on the processes of transition and transformation. Such stories can be instrumental in helping people to imagine what comes next, as life itself becomes invested with an ongoing sense of presence. Thérèse's narrative of continuity resonates with the story of an elderly woman I met late one afternoon. As soon as I entered the room, I noticed that the woman was very thin and frail, yet she had a beautiful smile and silver-white light sparkled in her dark brown eyes. As she told me:

> *The most wonderful thing for me right now*
> *Is to be with my husband.*
> *He's been deceased for a few years,*
> *But we were married for many decades.*
>
> *We really loved each other.*
> *We met at a little dance, in a little town,*
> *And I knew in an instant—like that—that he was the one.*
> *I knew, I think, because of his personality, and his kindness.*
> *He was a very caring man.*
> *He loved his children very much,*
> *And he loved life.*
> *He always said, "You make me happy."*
> *And I always said that to him, too.*
> *That feeling is beautiful.*
>
> *He's already here.*
> *I have seen him.*
> *I saw him in this room, at the corner, by the curtain,*
> *And I felt a tap on my shoulder.*
> *He looks the same as he did in life.*
> *It makes me feel so happy and wonderful.*
> *It's a soft, tender feeling.*
> *And, it's just there.*

Lyn Smallwood's illustration (Figure 34) depicts a frail elderly woman lying in bed, smiling at her husband who has passed away but who returns to her now. The vertical expanse of the white hospital bedsheet contrasts with the softly modulated pencil lines that demarcate the bouquet of flowers that bloom vibrantly on the adjacent tray table. Standing on the other side of the bouquet is a man with soft features and a glowing silhouette of silver-white light. While the man's form is less distinct than the woman's, there is a clear sense that these two people belong together.

When deceased loved ones appear as subtle living presences, people at the end of life recognize the part of themselves that cannot die. When we hear such stories, ordinary life can take on a new appearance, and the stories can serve as a life review for the living. After I read the narrative aloud, the woman closed the circle between death and life in a single gesture of saying goodbye and hello. As she told me:

> *When the time comes,*
> *I'm going to see even more bright light,*
> *And hopefully, I'll see him, too.*
> *And that completes the story.*

At its heart, this is a love story. It tells of beginnings, and ends, and beginning again. Paradoxically, *And That Completes the Story* tells a story that can never be completed, as the love continues on with a life of its own. That is why the love is seen as eternal, and why it is seen as sacred.

This sense of ongoing love enables us to face death and to see life. Or, put another way, you might say that as the woman saw the living image of her deceased husband and she felt the love they continued to share, she was encountering a rose from two gardens.

Notes

1. Regarding the phenomenon of individuals seeing visions of deceased relatives, friends, and other figures as they approach the end of life, see Janice Miner Holden, Bruce Greyson, and Debbie James, eds., *The Handbook of Near-Death Experiences: Thirty Years of Investigation* (Santa Barbara: Praeger Publishers, 2009), 231–32.
2. Quoted in *Story of a Soul*, 73, 81.
3. See the entry on "crypt" in *Webster's Seventh New Collegiate Dictionary*, 201.
4. The crypt is at once a place for containing presences and for knowing that the fullness of a person's life can never be fully contained. Just as these subjects will always exceed the language in which they are expressed, these themes resonate with key concepts that the philosopher Jacques Derrida explored in *The Gift of Death*. When commenting on the irreplaceable presence of the individual, Derrida observed that no one can die (or live) in the place of another. The conscious recognition of the intrinsic singularity of an individual life thus lies at the heart of the gift of death.
5. Quoted in *St. Thérèse of Lisieux*, 46.
6. Quoted in Thurston and Attwater, *Butler's Lives of the Saints*, vol. 4, 13–14.
7. See especially Lecture III, "The Reality of the Unseen," in William James, *The Varieties of Religious Experience: A Study in Human Nature* (1902; New York: Modern Library, 2002).
8. For a literature review and a rigorous critique of the term "hallucination" as a diagnostic category associated with deathbed visions and near-death experiences, see Allan Kellehear, "Unusual Perceptions at the End of Life: Limitations to the Diagnosis of Hallucinations in Palliative Medicine," *BMJ Supportive & Palliative Care* 7 (2017), 238–46. As Kellehear observes, describing these subjects as hallucinations promotes a stigmatizing approach that is often associated with psychopathology.
9. Allan Kellehear, *Visitors at the End of Life: Finding Meaning and Purpose in Near-Death Phenomena* (New York: Columbia University Press, 2020).
10. Kellehear, "Unusual perceptions at the end of life," 238–46.
11. Regarding these subjects, the physician Haider Warraich has observed that "the best way … of introducing religion and spirituality into a medical conversation remains controversial." Warraich emphasizes the importance of these topics *and* the difficulty many physicians face in bringing issues of religion and spiritual-

ity into healthcare discussions, particularly when confronting the end of life. As Warraich candidly notes, while "the cross section between religion, spirituality, and death is anathema to most physicians," not discussing "a patient's faith is tantamount to not treating them as a person." See Haider Warraich, *Modern Death: How Medicine Changed the End of Life* (New York: St. Martin's Press, 2017), 159, 168.

12. Quoted in *Story of a Soul*, 190–91.
13. Quoted in *Story of a Soul*, 191.

Note Regarding Issues of Confidentiality

The images appearing in this volume contain no recognizable likenesses that bear any resemblance to the individuals with whom I have worked. All of the illustrations were produced years after the visits occurred. With the exception of archival photographs of Thérèse of Lisieux, none of the visual works are based on photographic materials of any sort, nor do the images resemble any visual artworks now in the possession of surviving family members. In compliance with the federal standards of the United States Health Insurance Portability and Accountability Act (HIPAA), throughout this volume particular details relating to specific individuals have been altered or generalized so as to omit any identifiable data. These precautions are consistent with HIPAA compliance while preserving issues of confidentiality, particularly as specified under "The Privacy Rule," The Belmont Report, and the Department of Health and Human Services Office for Human Research Protections, including The Common Rule and subparts B, C, and D of the Health and Human Services specifications as outlined in the Code of Federal Regulations (CFR) at 45 CFR 164 and 165, which specifies the "safe harbor" method of de-identification. By adopting this approach, the stories are presented in such a way as to make the subjects visible *and* to acknowledge the legal and ethical frameworks that make such representations possible at all. Thus while the descriptions of encounters with patients and caregivers accurately reflect the nature of our interactions, and while the italicized texts are transcriptions of people's statements, these elements are generically worded, thus rendering the subjects anonymous. This project has been favorably reviewed by two independent Institutional Review Boards (IRBs) at Rice University and at the M.D. Anderson Cancer Center.

Bibliography

Primary Source

Archives of the Carmel of Lisieux, 37 Rue du Carmel, 14100, Lisieux, France.

Secondary Sources

American Heritage Dictionary of Indo-European Roots. Ed. Calvert Watkins. 2nd ed. Boston: Houghton Mifflin, 2000.

Attwater, Donald, ed. *A Dictionary of Saints.* London: Burns & Oates, 1958: 251.

Brennan, Marcia. *The Heart of the Hereafter: Love Stories from the End of Life.* Winchester, UK: Axis Mundi, 2014.

— *Life at the End of Life: Finding Words Beyond Words.* Bristol, UK: Intellect, 2017.

— *Put It On the Windowsill: An Italian-American Family Memoir.* Staffordshire, UK: Dark River, 2019.

Casarett, David. "Lessons in End-of-Life Care From the V.A." *The New York Times* (November 11, 2015): http://opinionator.blogs.nytimes. com/2015/11/11/lessons-in-end-of-life-care-from-the-v-a/?action=click &pgtype=Homepage&clickSource=story-heading&module=opinion-c-col-right-region&region=opinion-c-col-right-region&WT.nav=opinion-c-col-right-region&_r=0.

Charon, Rita. *Narrative Medicine: Honoring the Stories of Illness.* New York: Oxford University Press, 2006.

— et al. *The Principles and Practice of Narrative Medicine.* New York: Oxford University Press, 2016.

Chochinov, Harvey Max. *Dignity Therapy: Final Words for Final Days.* New York: Oxford University Press, 2012.

Derrida, Jacques. *The Gift of Death.* 2nd ed. Trans. David Wills. Chicago: University of Chicago Press, 2008.

Farmer, David Hugh. *The Oxford Dictionary of Saints.* 2nd ed. New York: Oxford University Press, 1987: 405–6.

Frohlich, Mary. *St. Thérèse of Lisieux: Essential Writings.* Maryknoll, NY: Orbis Books, 2007.

—. "The 'Thirst of Jesus' in the Vocations of Mother Teresa and Thérèse of Lisieux." *New Theology Review* 21, no. 4 (November 2008): 70–77.

Furlong, Monica. *Thérèse of Lisieux.* London: Virago, 1987.

Gawande, Atul. *Being Mortal: Medicine and What Matters in the End.* New York: Picador, 2017.

Görres, Ida. *The Hidden Face: A Study of St. Thérèse of Lisieux.* Freiburg im Breisgau: Herder Verlag, 1959.

Greeley, Andrew. *The Catholic Imagination.* Berkeley: University of California Press, 2000.

Green, James W. *Beyond the Good Death: The Anthropology of Modern Dying.* Philadelphia: University of Pennsylvania Press, 2008.

Hartley, Marsden. *On Art by Marsden Hartley.* Ed. Gail R. Scott. New York: Horizon Press, 1982.

Holden, Janice Miner, Bruce Greyson, and Debbie James. *The Handbook of Near-Death Experiences: Thirty Years of Investigation.* Santa Barbara: Praeger Publishers, 2009.

Howley, Lisa, Elizabeth Gaufberg, and Brandy King. *The Fundamental Role of the Arts and Humanities in Medical Education.* Washington, D.C.: Association of American Medical Colleges, 2020.

Institute of Medicine of the National Academies. *Dying in America: Improving Quality and Honoring Individual Preferences Near the End of Life.* New York: National Academies Press, 2014.

James, William. *The Varieties of Religious Experience: A Study in Human Nature.* New York: Modern Library, 2002.

Kaasa, Stein et al. "Integration of Oncology and Palliative Care: A Lancet Oncology Commission." *Lancet Oncology* 19 (November 1, 2018): e588–e653.

Kellehear, Allan. *The Inner Life of the Dying Person.* New York: Columbia University Press, 2014.

—. "Unusual Perceptions at the End of Life: Limitations to the Diagnosis of Hallucinations in Palliative Medicine." *BMJ Supportive & Palliative Care* 7 (2017): 238-46.

—. *Visitors at the End of Life: Finding Meaning and Purpose in Near-Death Phenomena.* New York: Columbia University Press, 2020.

Kleinman, Arthur. *The Illness Narratives: Suffering, Healing, and the Human Condition.* New York: Basic Books, 1988.

Lawton, Julia. *The Dying Process: Patients' Experiences of Palliative Care.* New York: Routledge, 2000.

Lisieux, Thérèse de. *St. Thérèse of Lisieux: Her Last Conversations.* Trans. John Clarke. Washington, D.C.: ICS Publications, 1977.

—. *Story of a Soul: The Autobiography of Saint Thérèse of Lisieux.* 3rd ed. Trans. John Clarke. Washington, D.C.: ICS Publications, 1996.

Marion, Jean-Luc. *God Without Being: Hors-Texte.* 2nd ed. Trans. Thomas A. Carlson. Chicago: University of Chicago Press, 2012.

—. *In the Self's Place: The Approach of Saint Augustine.* Trans. Jeffrey L. Kosky. Chicago: University of Chicago Press, 2012.

McBrien, Richard P. *The HarperCollins Encyclopedia of Catholicism.* San Francisco: HarperSanFrancisco, 1995: 1251–52.

Meltzer, Françoise and Jaś Elsner, eds. *Saints: Faith Without Borders.* Chicago: University of Chicago Press, 2011.

Morgan, David. *The Lure of Images: A History of Religion and Visual Media in America.* New York: Routledge, 2007.

National Academies of Sciences, Engineering, and Medicine. *The Integration of the Humanities and Arts with Sciences, Engineering, and Medicine in Higher Education: Branches of the Same Tree.* Washington, D.C.: The National Academies Press, 2018.

Nevin, Thomas R. *The Last Years of Saint Thérèse: Doubt and Darkness, 1895–1897.* New York: Oxford University Press, 2013.

—. *Thérèse of Lisieux: God's Gentle Warrior.* New York: Oxford University Press, 2006.

Orsi, Robert A. *Between Heaven and Earth: The Religious Worlds People Make and the Scholars Who Study Them.* Princeton: Princeton University Press, 2005.

—. *History and Presence.* Cambridge: Harvard University Press, 2016.

Oxford English Dictionary. 2nd ed. Oxford: Clarendon Press, 1989.

Remen, Rachel Naomi. *Kitchen Table Wisdom: Stories that Heal.* New York: Riverhead Books, 1996.

Robo, Etienne. *Two Portraits of St. Teresa of Lisieux.* Glasgow: Sands, 1955.

Rohrbach, Peter-Thomas. *The Search for Saint Thérèse.* Garden City, NY: Doubleday, 1961.

—. "Thérèse of Lisieux." *Encyclopedia of Religion.* 2nd ed. vol. 13. Ed. Lindsay Jones. Detroit: Macmillan Reference, 2005: 9155.

Sackville-West, Vita. *The Eagle and the Dove.* London: Pan Macmillan, 2011.

Saint Teresa. *Poems of St. Teresa, Carmelite of Lisieux, known as the 'Little Flower of Jesus'.* Grand Rapids, MI: Christian Classics Ethereal Library, n.d.

Saunders, Cicely, Mary Baines, and Robert Dunlop. *Living With Dying: A Guide to Palliative Care.* 3rd ed. New York: Oxford University Press, 1995.

Thurston, Herbert J. and Donald Attwater. "St. Teresa of Lisieux." *Butler's Lives of the Saints.* vol. 4. Westminster, MD: Christian Classics, 1990: 12–16.

Warraich, Haider. *Modern Death: How Medicine Changed the End of Life.* New York: St. Martin's Press, 2017.

Webster's Seventh New Collegiate Dictionary. Springfield, MA: Merriam, 1969.

Wright, Michael and David Clark. "Cicely Saunders and the Development of Hospice Palliative Care." *Religious Understandings of a Good Death in Hospice Palliative Care.* Ed. Harold Coward and Kelli I. Stajduhar. Albany: SUNY Press, 2012.

Index

www.ingramcontent.com/pod-product-compliance
Lightning Source LLC
Chambersburg PA
CBHW070910270326
41927CB00011B/2519